Cosmetic Patient Selection and Psychosocial Background

Panagiotis Milothridis

Cosmetic Patient Selection and Psychosocial Background

A Clinical Guide to Post-operative Satisfaction

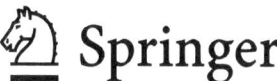 Springer

Panagiotis Milothridis
Thessaloniki
Greece

ISBN 978-3-030-44724-3   ISBN 978-3-030-44725-0   (eBook)
https://doi.org/10.1007/978-3-030-44725-0

This Springer imprint is published by the registered company Springer Nature Switzerland AG
The registered company address is: Gewerbestrasse 11, 6330 Cham, Switzerland

This book is dedicated to my beloved parents, Spiros and Vasiliki

Preface

As a plastic surgeon in private practice, I have noticed a portion of cosmetic patients with descent postoperative results who find it difficult to be happy with their new image. These unlucky patients cannot feel significant improvement in their self-esteem and quality of life, even if there may be an objectively fair result. But is it a matter of bad luck?

In fact, the problem in these cases has been my inability to understand the pure motivation of my patients and identify those who are not likely to benefit from the procedure. As doctors we all try to reach an excellent standard of clinical practice, but we generally neglect improving our communicational skills to achieve an optimal physician–cosmetic candidate relationship. The educational programs of the majority of medical schools also do not include lessons about patient selection in cosmetic medicine.

However, physicians who treat problematic patients suffer significant psychological and potentially financial burden. Medical litigation is on the rise against cosmetic doctors. Unhappy patients may also become aggressive and even violent toward their treating physician if they realize that their expectation differed from reality.

It is imperative to develop our skills to communicate and to better understand our patients. We have to learn how to approach the following questions: Why do our patients seek cosmetic procedures, while others with similar defects in appearance are not interested in altering them? How can I identify the potentially problematic patient? This book analyzes the psychosocial parameters of cosmetic candidates from a clinical perspective to assist physicians achieve advanced skills in patient selection during the preoperative consultation.

Thessaloniki, Greece   Panagiotis Milothridis

Contents

About the Author

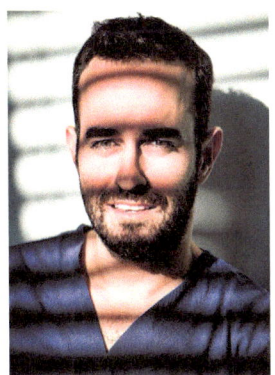

Panagiotis Milothridis was born in Kavala, a small town of northern Greece, in 1984. He studied Medicine in Democritus University of Thrace (D.u.Th.) and graduated in 2008. The decision to become a plastic surgeon was a one-way road. It was the artistic nature of the specialty along with the opportunity to improve someone's well-being that used to thrill him as a medical student. He completed his residency program in plastic surgery in Greece in 2017, and continued working as a fellow in facial plastic surgery in Istanbul, Turkey, in 2018. Now, he is a plastic surgeon in private practice owning two offices in Thessaloniki and Chios island in Greece. His humanitarian work consisted of a mission as a doctor without borders (MSF) to provide health care to refugees in Greece–Turkey borders and as a cleft surgeon in an Operation Smile (OS) mission in Madagascar to restore patients with cleft deformities. During the years of residency, he had two Masters of Science in Aristotle University of Thessaloniki (A.u.Th.) about Medical Research Methodology and Bioethics and Medical Law. During his bioethical studies, he realized that there should be a more defined strategy to select cosmetic patients, to achieve optimum postoperative benefit and minimize harm. At that time, he was named after a PhD in Medical School of A.u.TH. following 3 years of research over the psychosocial characteristics of cosmetic patients. Given the lack of evidence-based guidelines for cosmetic patient selection, his endeavors to develop a useful clinical tool for aesthetic practitioners led to the authorship of this book.

The Elective Nature of Cosmetic Medicine

1.1 Introduction

The history of beauty is as old as mankind itself—throughout history people have tried to improve their attractiveness and to enhance their beauty. Although great philosopher such as Plato or Immanuel Kant tried to define the term beauty, a universally valid definition remains elusive [1]. Nowadays, it is believed that key features such as clarity, symmetry, harmony, and vivid color are elements of an attractive and beautiful appearance.

Maybe more than men, women have the tendency to take care of their appearance and reverse the signs of aging. This is consistent with the strict social standards of female attractiveness. The shape of the so-called perfect woman has changed significantly over time. In the early 1900s, the ideal woman had either a voluptuous, round, full figure or she had a slim frame with larger breasts and hips [2]. These body types symbolized sexuality at that time. During the twentieth century, the ideal woman grew taller, her waist and hips became smaller, and her breasts became larger. Today, the ideal female figure is slim and muscular with large breasts, which naturally occur in a small percentage of women.

Therefore, people tend to seek either surgical or conservative cosmetic treatments to follow the beauty standards set by society. Cosmetic surgery is performed to reshape normal structures of the body in order to improve the patient's appearance and self-esteem in the absence of medical background such as disease or trauma. Despite the financial crisis of the last decade, cosmetic medicine industry keeps flourishing. According to 2018 ASPS Statistics Report [3], 16.5 billion US dollars was spent for 17,721,671 surgical and nonsurgical cosmetic procedures performed in 2018 in the USA. This number of procedures represents a 2% rise from 2017 and a 163% rise from 2000. Regarding surgical operations, breast augmentation was the most common with 313,000 procedures performed. The top five list also includes liposuction, nose reshaping, eyelid surgery, and tummy tuck.

The factors suggested to explain the rise in demand for cosmetic procedures include an increasing desire to appear youthful, social acceptability and increased

© Springer Nature Switzerland AG 2020
P. Milothridis, *Cosmetic Patient Selection and Psychosocial Background*,
https://doi.org/10.1007/978-3-030-44725-0_1

public awareness of CP, affordability, patient safety, and the introduction of minimally invasive procedures with shorter recovery times [4]. Minimally invasive procedures comprise a quick and efficient way to improve someone's appearance. In 2018, 15.9 million cosmetic minimally invasive procedures were performed which represents a 3% rise since 2017 and a 228% rise since 2000. It was also the year that marked the highest number of botulinum toxin type A injections to date with over 7.4 million injections. The top five list also includes soft tissue fillers (2.6 million), chemical peel (1.38 million), laser hair removal (1.0 million), and microdermabrasion (709,000).

Regarding gender, women represent 92% of all cosmetic patients. The age group that is more likely to undergo a cosmetic procedure is the 40–59-year-old patients (49%). Teenagers make up the least number of cosmetic procedures—only 1%. Some of the most common procedures for teens were nose reshaping, male breast reduction, ear surgery, laser hair removal, and laser skin resurfacing.

Mass media (magazines, movies, television, and the Internet) are influential promoters of beauty ideals. Unfortunately, the current images of beauty found in mass media are sometimes unrealistic, unattainable, and potentially unhealthy. These sociocultural influences interact with the physiological need to be attractive as part of the evolutionary theory and the sexual selection. They both lead to increased popularity of cosmetic procedures [5].

Physical image is taken into consideration during people's interactions. Abnormalities of body appearance can cause misidentification by the peer group [6]. For example, the large breasted woman may feel identified as a sexual object, the small breasted as unfeminine, the scarred face as threatening or criminal, and the wrinkled face as tired or old. These perceptions underline the significance of beauty in modern societies.

Despite their increasing popularity, not everyone benefits from cosmetic procedures. Certain psychosocial characteristics like body dysmorphic disorder (BDD) are associated with lower satisfaction and improvement in self-esteem and quality of life. Given that elective cosmetic surgery does not aim to cure disease or treat injury, physicians have to develop their clinical skills to identify the patients who will benefit the most from the procedures. Patient selection is an integral part of preoperative consultation.

1.2   Determinants of Beauty

Physical appearance plays a key role in evolutionary theory. According to Darwin, the ultimate goal of all species is reproduction [7]. Many physical characteristics have evolved in specific ways that make a given animal attractive and therefore promote reproduction. Birds with vivid colors are more likely to find a mate, even if they are more easily noted by predators. According to Darwin, sexual selection is the theory that certain physical characteristics have evolved because of reproductive rather than survival advantage.

This is also relevant for humans, as beauty plays an important role in the selection of human romantic and sexual partners. It is found that across 37 countries, both males and females prioritize physical attractiveness over personality traits such as dependability, emotional stability, and maturity in their choice of mates [8].

A youthful appearance also signals reproductive potential [9]. Ratings of youthfulness are highly correlated with ratings of attractiveness, typically declining with age particularly for women. Women are rated less feminine as they age, whereas men's ratings of masculinity do not change with age [10]. The value that people place on youthfulness is consistent with the sexual selection theory. Antiaging cosmetic treatments designed to restore an individual's facial appearance to a more youthful state, such as face-lifts and blepharoplasties, have long been considered some of the most popular procedures. Maybe Another indicator of beauty is bilateral symmetry. Studies of various animal species suggest that symmetrical animals are at a reproductive advantage compared to nonsymmetrical ones [11, 12]. Similarly, men and women with more symmetrical facial features are judged to be more attractive [13].

The ideal composite female face is petite with a mouth that is smaller than average but with full lips, a preadolescent jawline, and pronounced eyes and cheekbones [14]. Clear skin, bright eyes, and lustrous hair are also markers for beauty [8].

Regarding bodily norms, waist-hip ratio (WHR) is also thought to signal physical beauty for women [15]. WHR reflects the distribution of fat between the upper and lower body relative to the amount of abdominal fat. Healthy, fertile women typically have WHRs of 0.6 to 0.8. Studies support that men rate women with a low WHR (less than 0.8) as more attractive, healthier, and more feminine looking than women with a high WHR [16]. This can explain the statistical finding that liposuction which can alter WHR is one of the most popular cosmetic surgery procedures.

1.3 History of Cosmetic Procedures

People were involved in self-care since antiquity. The ancient Egyptians had been using animal oils, salt, alabaster, and sour milk to aesthetically improve their skin. Surgical techniques also have a long tradition. Over 2000 years ago, the forehead flap was used in India to reconstruct noses mutilated by war and criminal punishment. Either surgically or conservatively, people had been trying to improve physical appearance.

However, it was not until the late nineteenth century when the primary basis of cosmetic medicine was set and evolved to the modern standards of today.

At that time, it was established as an independent medical field. Dr. Edmund Saalfeld considered cosmetic medicine as the youngest primarily field of dermatology [17], as physicians of that time focused mainly on improving skin quality. In 1871, Tillbury Fox described the use of 20% phenol in order to lighten the skin, which became the first chemical peel. Paul G. Unna refined the technique of chemical peeling introducing salicylic acid, resorcinol, and trichloroacetic acid (TCA).

Safety of some procedures of the time used to be dubious. The first cosmetic doctors warned patients about the possible complications of treatments of the time. For example, facial enameling, a method originating from France, involved applying a heavy makeup paste composed by white lead pigment and other substances to the face. This reduced facial expressions and speech to a minimum. Early cosmetic doctors warned that this technique causes the skin to suffer substantially, thus only worsening the original condition [17]. They had the difficult task to examine the safety and efficacy of aesthetic procedures in favor of their patients' benefit.

Another procedure for removal of wrinkles that was popular in France in the nineteenth century was the so-called d'Arsonvalisation. It involved treatments with high-frequency alternating (Tesla) currents that would change direction over 100,000 times. Pashkis warned that this method would cause alopecia and loss of shine and force of the remaining hairs [18].

At that time, controlling emotional excesses was believed to be necessary to prevent aging. Excitement and anger would be avoided due to contraction of facial muscles. Sexual escapades were thought to contribute to premature aging by causing bloated features, sagging cheeks, and sunken eyes and were discouraged by charlatans [19].

Antiseptic surgery was developed in 1867 by the British surgeon Josef Lister. It resulted in fewer postoperative infections by using carbolic acid to sterilize instruments and to clean the surgical field. This increased safety led to novel cosmetic surgery treatments. In 1881, Robert T. Ely described the first otoplasty for protruding ears, and 6 years later John O. Roe performed the first subcutaneous rhinoplasty. At the end of the nineteenth century, Vincent Czerny introduced the first augmentation mammoplasty transplanting a lipoma of the patient.

The force of this desire for beauty was so great that even the outbreak of the First World War could not inhibit the rise of cosmetics. Not even the economic crisis of the mid-war turned people indifferent toward their physical appearance. Eventually, obsession with beauty spread from the upper to all classes leading to mass consumption of cosmetic services.

Cosmetic techniques evolved in consistency with beauty standards evolution. Aspects of beauty change over time because of sociocultural influences. At the start of the twentieth century, the "Gibson Girl" appeared, an icon combining fragile and delicate features with curvaceous breasts and hips. Women tried to mimic this style by many means such as the use of corsets [20].

The hourglass figures of Marilyn Monroe, as well as those of Jane Russell and Jane Mansfield, were the physical ideals of the 1950s [21]. These also inspired the production of the well-known doll Barbie. Monroe was photographed in 1953 for the first cover of the *Playboy* magazine, which has demonstrated beauty icons ever since.

During the 1960s, many beauty icons became less curvaceous [20]. That time dramatically thinner fashion icons, as the model Twiggy, became the new ideal. Although the superthin icon had faded during the 1970s, thinness has remained the characteristic of physical beauty. The majority of Miss America winners by this time had a body mass index (BMI) < 18.5, considered clinically underweight [22].

In the 1990s, two new physical characteristics have become the standards of female beauty. Muscular appearance with defined biceps, muscular legs, and "six pack" abdominal muscles in combination with large breasts was considered the new trend. This physical ideal is represented by the actress Pamela Anderson. The combination of thinness with the new characteristics of muscularity and large breasts rarely occurs in nature without cosmetic surgery and led to dramatic increase in breast augmentation procedures [5].

1.4 Cosmetic Medicine in the Twenty-First Century

Nowadays, access to cosmetic procedures is easier, and potential patients are better informed about them. Mass media (magazines, movies, television, and the Internet) are influential promoters of beauty ideals. Sometimes media images suggest that thinness and beauty is associated with success and popularity [23].

Cosmetic patients are also significantly influenced by the lifestyle and actions of celebrities. It is not unusual that they are presented in the preoperative consultation with photos of their idols to indicate their aesthetic requests. Celebrity influence can affect many aspects of consumer product choice, including technology, fashion, aesthetics, and healthcare.

This profound effect on general population is represented by the well-known example of Angelina Jolie's prophylactic mastectomy. Her announcement in *The New York Times* in May 2013 and the following increased popularity of BRCA1 and BRCA2 gene testing and risk-reducing mastectomy is now termed as the "Angelina Jolie" effect. It is the concept that high-profile celebrity announcements can have major, persistent influences on elective healthcare decisions by the general population [24].

Google Trends (GT) is a method of monitoring Internet search trends by analyzing the frequency of Google inquiries during a specific time period. Interest in plastic surgery and minimally invasive cosmetic procedures can be easily screened with the use of GT [25]. Google search terms "BRCA genes," "BRCA1," "BRCA2," "mastectomy," and "prophylactic mastectomy" demonstrated peak interest during the month of May 2013, following Angelina Jolie's announcement that she had undergone prophylactic mastectomy. This increased popularity has been also found in the long term as the search rates were significantly higher even years after the announcement. GT correlates significantly with actual healthcare practices, for example, increased BRCA testing and RRPM.

In accordance with Angelina Jolie, Kylie Jenner's announcement that she had undergone lip augmentation in May 2015 led to increased public interest in this minimally invasive cosmetic procedure. The increased popularity was also sustained in the long term. Similar effects were produced by April 2017 announcement of Caitlyn Jenner's gender-affirming surgery and February 2014 media attention given to Kim Kardashian's rumored buttock augmentation. Public announcements like Jolie's and the Kardashian family's have had lasting changes on public interest in healthcare and cosmetic medicine.

The evolution of image-centered social media has influenced people toward cosmetic medicine services. Easy editing of selfies on applications like Facetune and Snapchat has changed people's perception of beauty worldwide. In fact, people may seek cosmetic procedures so as to look better in selfies. Current data show that 55% of plastic surgeons report seeing patients who request surgery to improve their appearance in selfies, up from 42% in 2015 [26].

Excessive scrutiny of selfies is also changing the presenting concerns of patients. Prior to the popularity of selfies, the most common complaint of those requesting rhinoplasty was the hump of the dorsum of the nose. On the contrary, today, nasal and facial asymmetry is the most common complaint. Along with rhinoplasties, hair transplants and eyelid surgical procedures are also popular procedures to improve selfie appearance [27].

In the past, photo-editing technology was widely available only for celebrities. The appearance of models and actors was made perfect, and the general public was left to idolize their beauty. Thus, cosmetic patients used to bring photographs of celebrities to their consultations to better explain their desires. Nowadays, they are presented with filtered versions of themselves with fuller lips, bigger eyes, or a thinner nose. This new phenomenon called "Snapchat dysmorphia" is an alarming trend because filtered photographs may cross the border between reality and fantasy for these people.

Social media are currently used as a multipurpose tool for physician referral services, support groups, and disease education [28]. Similarly, cosmetic doctors use social media for communication with patients, practice recruitment, research, and professional image development.

Their professional site is also useful for them. Before choosing a cosmetic practice, patients are significantly more influenced by the relevant Web site (53%) than by any social media network [29]. A Web site allows for immediate access to in-depth content, an array of photographs, a library of videos, patient testimonials, blogs, articles, and links to other practice social media networks.

Regarding social media, cosmetic patients prefer the more easily digestible before-and-after photographs and information about the practice, along with the light-hearted excitement of contests for free products or treatments [30]. On the contrary, articles are the least favorite type of posts among cosmetic patients.

1.5 Is Every Cosmetic Doctor Obliged to Perform Any Procedure They Are Asked to?

Patient selection is an internal part of cosmetic healthcare. Aesthetic doctors have the right to refuse to be involved in treatments that either may not be beneficial for their patients or are believed to be morally controversial. Conscientious objection can be broadly defined as the refusal by a healthcare practitioner to perform a legal medical activity considered beneficial by the patient [31].

Cosmetic surgery has been occasionally used for artistic purposes. Stelarc is an Australian artist who believes that human body is obsolete. He has tried to show that being human is not determined merely by biological structures rather than the technology that is plugged into someone's body [32]. In 2007, he had a prosthetic ear inserted in his arm and declared that it took him 10 years to find doctors willing to perform such intervention.

Others seek cosmetic surgery for funny and trivial reasons. An example is Dennis Avner, also known as the Stalking Cat, who underwent 14 operations in order to look like a feline [33]. Among other procedures, he underwent bifurcation of the upper lip and a septum relocation aimed at making his nose look flatter. An alternative trend has been to use cosmetic surgery for political reasons. Morgan suggested that in order to destabilize the current chauvinist standard of beauty, women could undergo "uglifying" cosmetic surgery, including bleaching one's hair white, applying wrinkle-inducing creams, "wrinkle creams," having one's face and breasts surgically pulled down (rather than lifted), and having wrinkles sewn and carved into one's skin [34].

Sometimes non-Caucasian patients want to undergo cosmetic procedures in order to look Caucasian. If a black person wants to undergo an operation to change his/her skin color, it may be because this race is discriminated against rather than because of a genuine desire to look more attractive. Such intervention may benefit individual patients, yet it would harm society at large.

If physicians decide that the cosmetic procedure will not be beneficial for their patients in terms of postoperative satisfaction, improvement in quality of life or self-esteem is justified to refuse to offer their services. Patients' motivation should also be examined.

1.6   Conclusion

Cosmetic medicine techniques have been widely used to improve someone's appearance. Combining the past, present, and future of cosmetic medicine allows doctors to incorporate this perspective and ultimately to deliver better patient care. Additionally, better understanding of the motivations of modern patients allows for optimal selection during preoperative consultation.

References

1. Krueger N, Luebberding S, Sattler G, Hanke CW, Alexiades-Armenakas M, Sadick N. The history of aesthetic medicine and surgery. J Drugs Dermatol. 2013;12(7):737–42.
2. Gordon KH, Castro Y, Sitnikov L, Holm-Denoma JM. Cultural body shape ideals and eating disorder symptoms among White, Latina, and Black college women. PsycNET. Accessed 6 Sep 2018.
3. ASPS Statistics 2018. https://www.plasticsurgery.org/documents/News/Statistics/2018/plastic-surgery-statistics-full-report-2018.pdf.

4. Crockett RJ, Pruzinsky T, Persing JA. The influence of plastic surgery "reality TV" on cosmetic surgery patient expectations and decision making. Plast Reconstr Surg. 2007;120:316–24.
5. Sarwer DB, Magee L, Clark V. Physical appearance and cosmetic medical treatments: physiological and sociocultural influences. J Cosmet Dermatol. 2003;2(1):29–39.
6. Khoo CTK. Cosmetic surgery e where does it begin? Br J Plast Surg. 1982;35:277e80.
7. Darwin C. The origin of species. New York: Books, Inc.; 1900.
8. Buss DM, Abbot M, Angleitner A. International preferences in selecting mates: a study of 37 cultures. J Cross Cultural Psychol. 1990;35:5–47.
9. Symons D. The evolution of human sexuality. New York: Oxford University Press; 1979.
10. Deutsch FM, Zalenski CM, Clark ME. Is there a double standard of aging? J Appl Soc Psychol. 2002;16:771–85.
11. Moller AP. Female swallow preferences for symmetrical male sexual ornaments. Nature. 1992;357:238–40.
12. Petrie M, Halliday TR, Sanders C. Peahens prefer peacocks with elaborate trains. Anim Behav. 1991;41:323–31.
13. Gangestad SW, Thornhill R, Yeo R. Facial attractiveness, developmental stability and fluctuating asymmetry. Ethol Sociobiol. 1994;15:73–85.
14. Johnston VS, Franklin M. Is the beauty in the eye of the beholder? Ethol Sociobiol. 1991;14:183–99.
15. Singh D. Adaptive significance of female physical attractiveness: role of waist-to-hip ratio. J Pers Soc Psychol. 1993;65:456–66.
16. Singh D. Female judgement of male attractiveness and desirability for relationships: role of waist-to-hip ratio and financial status. J Pers Soc Psychol. 1995;69:1089–101.
17. Kosmetik SE. Ein Leitfaden für praktische Ärzte. Berlin: Springer; 1908.
18. Paschkis H. Kosmetik für Ärzteumgearbuverm. Wien, Alfred Hölder: Auflage; 1905.
19. Lorand A. Die Kosmetik des Alterns. In: Joseph M, editor. Handbuch der Kosmetik. Leipzig: von Veit & Comp; 1912. p. 105–15.
20. Mazur A. U.S. trends in feminine beauty and overadaptation. J Sex Res. 1986;22:281–303.
21. Fallon A. Culture in the mirror: sociocultural determinants of body image. In: Cash TF, Pruzinsky T, editors. Body images: development, deviance and change. New York: The Guilford Press; 1990. p. 80–109.
22. Rubinstein S, Caballero B. Is Miss America an undernourished role model? JAMA. 2000;283:1569.
23. Wolf N. The beauty myth. New York: William Morrow; 1991.
24. Tijerina JD, Morrison SD, Nolan IT, Parham MJ, Richardson MT, Nazerali R. Celebrity influence affecting public interest in plastic surgery procedures: Google trends analysis. Aesthet Plast Surg. 2019;43(6):1669–80.
25. Vasconcellos-Silva PR, Carvalho DB, Trajano V, de La Rocque LR, Sawada AC, Juvanhol LL. Using Google trends data to study public interest in breast cancer screening in Brazil: why not a Pink February? JMIR Public Health Surveill. 2007;3(2):e17.
26. American Academy of Facial Plastic and Reconstructive Surgery. Annual Survey Statistics, 2018. https://www.aafprs.org/media/stats_polls/m_stats.html. Published January 29, 2018. Accessed 06 Mar 2018.
27. Özgür E, Muluk NB, Cingi C. Is selfie a new cause of increasing rhinoplasties? Facial Plast Surg. 2017;33(4):423–7.
28. Ross NA, Todd Q, Saedi N. Patient seeking behaviors and online personas. Dermatol Surg. 2015;41(2):269–76.
29. Sorice SC, Li AY, Gilstrap J, Canales FL, Furnas HJ. Social media and the plastic surgery patient. Plast Reconstr Surg. 2017;140(5):1047–56.
30. Pulizzi J. What is content marketing? In: Pulizzi J, editor. Epic content marketing: how to tell a different story, breakthrough the clutter, & win more customers by marketing less. New York: McGraw-Hill Education; 2014. p. 3–11.

31. Minerva F. Cosmetic surgery and conscientious objection. J Med Ethics. 2017;43(4):230–3.
32. http://edition.cnn.com/2015/08/13/arts/stelarc-ear-arm-art/. Accessed 10 Jul 2016.
33. https://en.wikipedia.org/wiki/Stalking_Cat. Accessed 10 Jul 2016.
34. Morgan KP. Women and the knife: cosmetic surgery and the colonization of women's bodies. Hypatia. 1991;6:25–53. 46

Postoperative Benefit of Cosmetic Procedures

2.1 Introduction

The modern perception of health does not simply refer to the absence of physical or mental disease. The definition of health by the World Health Organization (WHO) involves complete physical, psychological, and social well-being rather than just the absence of disease [1]. This is relevant with the ultimate goal of cosmetic procedures, as they are performed to improve someone's psychosocial status by improving their appearance.

In the absence of physical dysfunction, elective cosmetic surgery is performed to improve someone's well-being by increasing body image, self-esteem, and postoperative satisfaction. The public often perceive cosmetic surgery to be trivial and of lower priority compared with other medical interventions [2]. Additionally, third-party payers in most healthcare systems do not cover for cosmetic surgery expenses. Postoperative benefit of elective plastic surgery is usually underestimated.

However, patients feel more confident and more satisfied with their appearance, and they demonstrate increased psychological well-being following the aesthetic procedure. Cosmetic medicine seems to reduce the occurrence of both negative emotional and behavioral body image experiences. Even though postoperative benefit seems to be subjective, it is objectively quantifiable with patient-reported questionnaires.

2.2 Quantification of Benefit in Cosmetic Medicine

There are certain psychosocial parameters that comprise the postoperative benefit following cosmetic procedures. These are:

- Satisfaction with overall appearance or with a specific body part.
- Health-related quality of life.
- Sexual life.

© Springer Nature Switzerland AG 2020
P. Milothridis, *Cosmetic Patient Selection and Psychosocial Background*,
https://doi.org/10.1007/978-3-030-44725-0_2

- Mental health.
- Self-esteem.
- Body image.

2.3   Postoperative Satisfaction

Cosmetic patients are usually motivated to undergo a cosmetic procedure because of dissatisfaction with their overall appearance or a specific feature [3]. Therefore, a primary measurement of postoperative benefit is patient satisfaction [4–8]. Satisfaction is referred either to the general appearance or the body part being operated and is found to be improved even 5 years following the cosmetic procedure [9].

2.4   Health-Related Quality of Life

Quality of life (QoL or QOL) is the self-assessment of someone's well-being or lack thereof. It is a subjective multidimensional concept that defines a standard level for emotional, physical, material, and social well-being. It serves as a reference against which an individual or society can measure the different domains of one's own life.

It observes life satisfaction, including everything from physical health, family, education, employment, wealth, safety, security to freedom, religious beliefs, and the environment. According to the World Health Organization (WHO), quality of life is defined as "the individual's perception of their position in life in the context of the culture and value systems in which they live and relation to their goals."

2.4.1   Quality of Life Assessment

The Short Form 36 (SF-36) is a 36-item patient-reported survey of health-related quality of life. It consists of eight scaled scores, which are the weighted sums of the questions in their section. Each scale is directly transformed into a 0–100 scale on the assumption that each question carries equal weight. The lower the score, the poorest the QoL. The eight sections are vitality, physical functioning, bodily pain, general health perceptions, physical role functioning, emotional role functioning, social role functioning, and mental health [10].

The Glasgow Benefit Inventory (GBI) is an 18-item validated, generic patient-recorded outcome measure widely used in otorhinolaryngology to report change in quality of life post-intervention [11].

The Moorehead-Ardelt Quality of Life Questionnaire was initially developed and incorporated into the Bariatric Analysis and Reporting Outcome System Questionnaire for the evaluation of changes after bariatric surgery. It evaluates QoL on five domains: self-esteem, physical activity, social life, work conditions, and sexual activity. For each question, no changes after surgical intervention are scored by no points, improvements give partial positive points, and the negative effects diminish the total score, respectively. The questionnaire has a rating scale ranging from −3 (greatly diminished result) to 3 (greatly improved result) [12].

2.4.2 Postoperative Benefit in QoL

Most studies examining quality of life following cosmetic surgery focus on breast reduction. At baseline, all studies reported worse HRQL than population norms across most domains, while postoperatively they reported improvement equaling or surpassing population norms, particularly in the physical domains of HRQL [13]. Patients underwent moderate to large improvement for all dimensions of the SF-36: the greater improvement was in pain dimension, followed by great improvement in physical function.

Breast reduction patients are more broadly impaired than groups requesting other cosmetic procedures and so gain more from surgery. The benefits observed for SF-36 scores in breast reduction patients are of similar magnitude to those observed in patients experiencing improvements from a range of other hospital, medical, and surgical interventions, for example, peptic ulcer, rheumatoid arthritis, gall stones, and inguinal hernia [14].

Another study [15] reported the changes in HRQL of patients undergoing various procedures (breast reduction, breast reconstruction, other breast surgery, pinnaplasty, rhinoplasty, and abdominoplasty). All groups reported improvements in some aspect of social and/or psychological functioning or in the perception of health as in the case of rhinoplasty patients. The changes were small to moderate in size with the exception of breast reduction patients who underwent moderate to large change on all health status measures. In any case, the postoperative scores are within the range and more favorable than those of the general population. The group that showed the least difference in health status before and after surgery compared to the general population was the breast reconstruction patients.

Medial thighplasty also seems to improve the quality of life of patients in five domains of the Moorehead-Ardelt QoL Questionnaire. This procedure improved self-esteem in 90.5% of patients, physical status in 85.7% of patients, social life in 85.7% of patients, and labor in 76.5% of patients. Interestingly, no improvement was shown in sexual activity [16]. It facilitates the wearing of clothing, reduces the friction of thighs, and therefore allows improved walking in a global manner. Negative effects in QoL are associated with postoperative complication such as lymphedema.

Another study showed that all four domains of the Body-QoL tool were significantly better after body contouring surgery, both short and long term ($p < 0.0001$). BCS improves QoL by enhancing self-image, increasing self-esteem, reducing physical symptoms, and providing other favorable effects [17].

Analysis of the data of 90 patients who underwent rhinoplasty showed also significant improvement in quality of life [18]. McKienan et al. specified that surgery for aesthetic reason results in greater improvement than for functional reasons, while when both aesthetic and functional reasons combined, the level of benefit in quality of life is the highest [19].

2.5   Sexual Life

Sexual life is an important domain of life providing pleasure and psychological well-being. Dissatisfaction with appearance may negatively affect someone's sexual life, and cosmetic procedures seem to improve it. More precisely, a better perception of body/face, confidence, and attractiveness can result in an improved sexual life. Stofman et al. studied 70 female patients and showed that 70% testified that their sex life has been enhanced following cosmetic surgery. More than 30% of breast patients and 50% of body patients reported an enhanced ability to achieve orgasm [20]. In another study of 73 breast augmentation patients, 71% stated an increased sexuality after surgery [21].

2.6   Mental Health

Even though cosmetic procedures are not indicated to cure psychological disorders, it seems that they alleviate certain symptoms and improve mental health, especially in breast reduction patients. Commonly used questionnaires are Hospital Anxiety and Depression Score (HADS) and the General Health Questionnaire (GHQ).

HADS was originally developed by Zigmond and Snaith in 1983 and is commonly used to determine the levels of anxiety and depression that an individual experiences. It is a 14-item scale, seven referring to anxiety and seven to depression. At first it was created to evaluate anxiety and depression in people with physical illness, but it is also used in general population. A cutoff score of 8/21 is used for diagnosis [22].

The General Health Questionnaire (GHQ) is a screening device for identifying minor psychiatric disorders in general population and within community or nonpsychiatric clinical settings such as primary care or general outpatients. Lower scores indicate better psychological functioning. A case on the GHQ-28 is a score greater than 4 out of a possible 28 and is indicative of possible nonpsychotic psychiatric disturbance. A study reported that 30.1% of cosmetic patients scored as a case before surgery. After treatment, the proportion of cases fell to 17.7%. This is found to be the norm in general population. The breast reduction group had the highest proportion of cases preoperatively and lowest proportion postoperatively and was the only group for which the change proved to be statistically significant [15].

2.7   Self-Esteem

Self-esteem is someone's subjective evaluation of their own worth. It develops in accordance with someone's experiences in life. Unconditional love from parents during childhood and authoritative and permissive parenting style primarily allow for normal self-esteem development.

Individuals with high self-esteem are more extroverted, emotionally stable, and conscientious. On the contrary, people with low self-esteem occasionally have

Table 2.1 Characteristics of people with a healthy level of self-esteem

They trust their own values and defend them when finding opposition
They collaborate well with others and resist being manipulated
They consider themselves equal to others, unlike narcissists who have feelings of grandiosity
They enjoy a great variety of activities
They are sensitive to feelings and needs of others
They trust their ability to solve problems and can work toward this direction
They learn from the past and plan for the future

Table 2.2 Characteristics of people with low self-esteem

They are dissatisfied with life
They tend to constantly criticize themselves, but they are hypersensitive to criticism by others with feelings of being attacked
They have the need to please anyone
They are pessimists with general negative outcome
They suffer from chronic indecision being afraid of making mistakes
They are perfectionists, but when perfection is not achieved, they feel frustrated

feelings of shame, such as in cases of social evaluated poor performances [23]. The characteristics of individuals with normal and low self-esteem are presented in Tables 2.1 and 2.2.

Self-esteem is typically assessed using self-report inventories. One of the most widely used is the Rosenberg scale, which is a 10-item Likert scale ranging from 4 (strongly agree) to 1 (strongly disagree). It is designed to measure subjects' self-concept. Higher scores indicate higher self-esteem. It is brief and widely used in cosmetic surgery studies. An alternative measure is the Coopersmith's inventory.

In medical literature, there are seven studies evaluating any change in self-esteem following CS. Breast reduction patients reported significant improvement in self-esteem and in psychological well-being (**General Health Questionnaire**) 6 months postoperatively [14]. Another qualitative study showed improved self-image and self-confidence after 2 years as shown in the Rosenberg scores. In their interview, the majority of breast reduction patients explained that their improved appearance led to enhanced self-confidence because they "look normal" and have a greater choice of attractive clothes and underwear. They also claim that their personal life as well as their professional relationships improved, and as a result they have enhanced relationships with partners and friends as well as better work perspective [24].

A study that examined changes after various procedures concludes that the greatest amount of change, which ranged from moderate to large, was experienced in self-esteem [15].

A prospective study of rhinoplasty patients showed significant improvement in the rating of self-esteem. Both the overall score and the individual subcomponents showed significant improvements at the long-term follow-up as compared with initial levels. Remarkably, changes were obvious at the 1-week postsurgical point. In specific, feelings of approval by others, contentment, and worthiness or feelings of personal significance and the value of existence were noted [25]. However, no changes were seen among abdominoplasty patients regarding their general psychosocial functioning (self-esteem, satisfaction with life, or social anxiety) [26].

In general, a moderate to large postoperative effect on self-esteem is seen after most procedures. A common limitation of most studies is that they have short follow-up periods. This may cause short-term cognitive dissonance effects of surgery [27]. Cognitive dissonance is scored according to what someone expects preoperatively about the result of the procedure.

2.8   Body Image

Body image is a person's perception of the appearance of their own body. It refers to the sum total of conscious and unconscious attitudes toward our own bodies. It involves how an individual evaluates themselves compared to the standards set by society. There is developmental as well as sociocultural influence on body image.

Developmental influence	It refers to childhood and adolescent experiences
Sociocultural influence	It refers to the interaction and effect that social and cultural standards and mass media portrayal of beauty have on the person

The overall body image is a psychological entity, which is comprised of a perceptual and a dimensional dimension [28]. Perceptual body image is the dimension that refers to how accurately individuals evaluate their body, whereas the attitudinal dimension is referred to individuals' beliefs and feelings about their physical appearance. Attitudinal body image can be further divided into two components, orientation and evaluation.

Body image orientation	Refers to the degree of importance the individuals place on their appearance
Body image evaluation	Refers to how satisfied they are with their body

Disoriented view of one's shape creates negative body image. Sufferers often feel ashamed and believe that others are more attractive. This could possibly lead to eating disorders, isolation, and mental illness. Its extreme form is body dysmorphic disorder, a mental disease characterized by the obsessive idea that a body part is severely flawed. On the contrary, individuals who evaluate highly their appearance are positive and satisfied.

Regarding body image orientation, people who are highly oriented place much importance on their appearance and engage in extensive grooming, while lower individuals with lower body image orientation are apathetic about their appearance and do not expect much effort to "look good."

On the contrary, positive body image consists of the true perception of someone's appearance. Cosmetic surgery is frequently described as body image surgery, and enhancing body image is considered to be a major motivation for seeking surgery.

2.8.1   Measurement Tools

Multidimensional Body-Self Relations Questionnaire (MBSRQ) is a widely used, self-report measurement tool of several aspects of body image of persons 15 years of age or older [29]. It consists of 69 items divided into 10 subscales that assess both individuals' investment in and satisfaction with their appearance, fitness, health, illness, and weight. It consists of the following subscales: appearance evaluation, appearance orientation, fitness evaluation, fitness orientation, health evaluation, health orientation, illness orientation, body area satisfaction, overweight preoccupation, and self-classified weight.

The first 57 items are answered on a five-point Likert scale from 1 (definitely disagree) to 5 (definitely agree). Higher scores mean greater investment or satisfaction with the specific domain. Items 61 to 69, representing the body area dissatisfaction subscale, use a five-point Likert scale indicating how dissatisfied or satisfied a person is with his or her body, with choices ranging from 1 (very dissatisfied) to 5 (very satisfied). The separate subscales can be evaluated either jointly or independently [30].

The Body Dysmorphic Disorder Examination Self-Report is a measure of body image dissatisfaction focused on a specific physical feature [31]. This is used as a diagnostic tool for BDD. Respondents rank the five features in their appearance with which they are most dissatisfied. They also answer questions on scales from 1 to 6 that assess preoccupation and negative evaluation of appearance, excessive importance of appearance, avoidance of activities and places, and body camouflaging.

The Body Satisfaction Scale (BSS) is a simple self-report questionnaire which was revised to record body image disturbances in subjects with eating disorders. The scale consists of a list of 16 parts, half involving the head (head, face, jaw, teeth, nose, mouth, eyes, and ears) and the other half involving the body (shoulders, neck, breasts, abdomen, arms, hands, legs, and feet). Respondents are asked to rate satisfaction/dissatisfaction with each of these body parts on a seven-point scale [32]. In medical literature, there are several studies comparing body image before and after CS. Three of them study the benefit of breast reduction over body image [33–35].

Body image evaluation was found to be lower in patients with macromastia and increased following surgery. There was no evidence of a shift in dissatisfaction to other parts of the body, but, rather, the opposite occurred with women reporting greater satisfaction with the rest of their bodies. Sarwer et al. [36] reported that following cosmetic surgery, women experience significant improvements in body image dissatisfaction with a specific feature altered. Postoperatively, patients reported less embarrassment about the feature when other people's attention was drawn there during social situations. The amount of time they are upset about the feature and the number of days they camouflaged the feature with clothing or makeup decreased significantly. However, authors could not generalize this effect to the overall body image.

Multidimensional Body-Self Relations Questionnaire and the Situational Inventory of Body Image Dysphoria [26] revealed significant improvements in body image outcome, including positive changes in patients' evaluations of overall appearance of abdominoplasty patients. Similar improvements in postoperative body satisfaction and evaluation of their appearance were reported for breast augmentation patients [37]. The abovementioned findings suggest that the negative body image symptoms, thoughts, feelings, and behaviors should be alleviated postoperatively.

2.9   Conclusion

Patients benefit from cosmetic procedures in terms of improvement of their psychosocial well-being. Health-related quality of life, self-esteem, body image, and mental health are the main parameters improved following cosmetic procedures. These are quantifiable via validated clinical tools. Cosmetic physicians have the task to identify the patients who will benefit the most.

References

1. World Health Organization. Constitution of the World Health Organization as adopted by the International Health Conference, New York, 19–22 June 1946; signed on 22 July 1946 by the representatives of 61 States (Official Records of the World Health Organization, no. 2, p. 100) and entered into force on 7 April 1948. In Grad, Frank P. The Preamble of the Constitution of the World Health Organization. Bull World Health Organ. 2002;80(12):982.
2. Bowling A, Jacobson B, Southgate L. Explorations in consultations of the public and health professionals on priority setting in an inner London health district. Soc Sci Med. 1993;37:851–7.
3. Alsarraf R, Larrabee WF Jr, Anderson S, Murakami CS, Johnson CM Jr. Measuring cosmetic facial plastic surgery outcomes: A pilot study. Arch Facial Plast Surg. 2001;3:198–201.
4. Rhee JS, McMullin BT. Outcome measures in facial plastic surgery: patient-reported and clinical efficacy measures. Arch Facial Plast Surg. 2008;10:194–207.
5. Kim JY, Cha MJ, Kwon SS, Kim DK. Factors that contribute to disagreement in satisfaction between surgeons and patients after corrective septorhinoplasty. Am J Rhinol Allergy. 2017;31:416–9.
6. Knorr NJ, Edgerton MT, Hoopes JE. The "insatiable" cosmetic surgery patient. Plast Reconstr Surg. 1967;40:285–9.
7. Nouraei SA, Pulido MA, Saleh HA. Impact of rhinoplasty on objective measurement and psychophysical appreciation of facial symmetry. Arch Facial Plast Surg. 2009;11:198–202.
8. Münker R. Facial profile correction and nasal appearance. Facial Plast Surg. 1995;11:138–58.
9. Von Soest T, Kvalem IL, Skolleborg KC, Roald HE. Psychosocial changes after cosmetic surgery: a 5-year follow-up study. Plast Reconstr Surg. 2011;128(3):765–72.

10. Rudolph C, Hladik C, Stroup DF, Frank K, Gotkin RH, Dayan SH, Patel A, Cotofana S. Are cosmetic procedures comparable to antidepressive medication for quality-of-life improvements? A systematic review and controlled meta-analysis. Facial Plast Surg. 2019;35(5):549–58.
11. Robinson K, Gatehouse S, Browning GG. Measuring patient benefit from otorhinolaryngological surgery and therapy. Ann Otol Rhinol Laryngol. 1996;105:415–22.
12. Moorehead MK, Ardelt-Gattinger E, Lechner H, Oria HE. The validation of the Moorehead-Ardelt Quality of Life Questionnaire II. Obes Surg. 2003;13:684–92.
13. Cook S, Rosser R, Salmon P. Is cosmetic surgery an effective psychotherapeutic intervention? A systematic review of the evidence. J Plast Reconstr Aesthetic Surg. 2006;59(11):1133–51.
14. Klassen A, Fitzpatrick R, Jenkinson C, Goodacre T. Should breast reduction surgery be rationed? A comparison of the health status of patients before and after treatment: postal questionnaire survey. BMJ. 1996;313(7055):454–7.
15. Klassen A, Jenkinson C, Fitzpatrick R, Goodacre T. Patients' health related quality of life before and after aesthetic surgery. Br J Plast Surg. 1996;49(7):433–8.
16. Bertheuil N, Thienot S, Chaput B, Varin A, Watier E. Quality of life assessment after medial thighplasty in patients following massive weight loss. Plast Reconstr Surg. 2015;135(1):67–73.
17. Suijker J, Troncoso E, Pizarro F, Montecinos S, Villarroel G, Erazo C, Danilla S. Long-term quality of life outcomes after body contouring surgery: phase IV results for the body-QoL cohort. Aesthet Surg J. 38(3):279–88.
18. Niehaus R, Kovacs L, Machens HG, Herschbach P, Papadopulos N. Quality of life – changes after rhinoplasty. Facial Plast Surg. 2017;33(05):530–6.
19. McKieman DC, Banfield G, Kumar R, Hinton AE. Patient benefit from functional and cosmetic rhinoplasty. Clin Otolaryngol Allied Sci. 2001;26(1):50–2.
20. Stofman GM, Neavin TS, Ramineni PM, Alford A. Better sex from the knife? An intimate look at the effects of cosmetic surgery on sexual practices. Aesthet Surg J. 2006;26(01):12–7.
21. Papadopoulos N, Totis A, Kiriakidis D, Mavroudis M, Henrich G, Papadopoulos O. Quality of life, personality changes, self-esteem, and emotional stability after breast augmentation. Eur J Plast Surg. 2014;37(09):479–88.
22. Bjelland I, Dahl AA, Haug TT, Neckelmann D. The validity of the hospital anxiety and depression scale. An updated literature review. J Psychosom Res. 2002;52(2):69–77.
23. Gruenewald TL, Kemeny ME, Aziz N, Fahey JL. Acute threat to the social self: shame, social self-esteem, and cortisol activity. Psychosom Med. 2004;66(6):915–24.
24. Shakespeare V, Postle K. A qualitative study of patients' views on the effects of breast-reduction surgery: a 2-year follow-up survey. Br J Plastic Surgery. 1999;52(3):198–204.
25. Sheard C, Jones NS, Qurashi MS, Herbert M. A prospective study of the psychological effects of rhinoplasty. Clin Otolaryngol. 1996;21(3):232–6.
26. Bolton MA, Pruzinsky T, Cash TF, Persing JA. Measuring outcomes in plastic surgery: body image and quality of life in abdominoplasty patients. Plast Reconst Surg. 2003;112(2):619–25.
27. Cook S, Rosser R, Salmon P. Is cosmetic surgery an effective psychotherapeutic intervention? A systematic review of the evidence. J Plast Reconstr Aesthet Surg. 2006;59(11):1133–51.
28. Cash TF. Body-image attitudes: evaluation, investment, and affect. Percept Mot Skills. 1994;78:1168–70.
29. Brown TA, Cash TF, Mikulka PJ. Attitudinal body-image assessment: factor analysis of the body-self relations questionnaire. J Pers Assess. 1990;55:135.
30. Cash TF. User's Manual for the Multidimensional Body–Self Relations Questionnaire. Accessed Jan 2005 at www.body-images.com.
31. Rosen JC, Reiter J. Development of the body dysmorphic disorder examination. Behav Res Ther. 1996;34:755.
32. Slade PD, Dewey ME, Newton T, Brodie D, Kiemle G. Development and preliminary validation of the body satisfaction scale (BSS). Psychol Health. 1990;4:213–20.
33. Faria FS, Guthrie E, Bradbury E, et al. Psychosocial outcome and patient satisfaction following breast reduction surgery. Br J Plast Surg. 1999;52:448–52.
34. Collins ED, Kerrigan CL, Kim M, et al. The effectiveness of surgical and non-surgical interventions in relieving the symptoms of macromastia. Plast Reconstr Surg. 2002;109:1556–66.

35. Kerrigan CL, Schwarz G, Charbonneau R. Measuring quality of life in women undergoing surgery for breast hypertrophy. Can J Plast Surg. 2001;9:221–5.
36. Sarwer DB, Wadden TA, Whtaker LA. An investigation of changes in body image following cosmetic surgery. Plast Reconstr Surg. 2002;109(1):363–9.
37. Banbury J, Yetman R, Lucas A, Papy F, Graves K, Zins JE. Prospective analysis of subpectoral breast augmentation: sensory changes, function, and body image. Plast Reconstr Surg. 2004;113:701–7.

Cosmetic Medicine: Are All People Equally Prone to Be Interested in It?

3

Definitions
The "Angelina Jolie effect" is the concept that high-profile celebrity announcements can have major, persistent influences on elective health-care decisions by the general population.

3.1 Introduction

The number of cosmetic procedures performed is constantly increasing. Beauty in modern cultures is defined by mass media through television and magazines. The perfect career, family, and social status all correlate with an impeccable physical appearance. Despite any financial crisis, cosmetic medicine industry keeps flourishing. According to the 2018 ASPS Statistics Report [1], 16.5 billion US dollars was spent for 17.721.671 surgical and nonsurgical cosmetic procedures performed in 2018 in the USA. People seek surgical treatments to improve defects in their appearance and to reverse the signs of time.

Minimally invasive cosmetic techniques are also a simple and quick way to freshen up the face and body with minimal cost and recovery time. Their popularity is further supported by the image-centered social media and smartphone applications like Snapchat. Edited photographs with filters present an improved version of people's face and motivate them to seek cosmetic services.

Physical appearance plays an important role in everyday social interactions. This may influence someone's motivation to pursue cosmetic medical treatments. Increase in self-confidence seems to be the primary motive. Most patients seek nonsurgical cosmetic procedures to look younger or fresher (83.4%) and to have clear skin (81.4%). They want to feel more attractive mainly for themselves (88.5%) rather than for others (64.4%) [2].

© Springer Nature Switzerland AG 2020
P. Milothridis, *Cosmetic Patient Selection and Psychosocial Background*,
https://doi.org/10.1007/978-3-030-44725-0_3

Additionally, the impact of social networks in someone's desire to look nice is also significant. Looking better in photographs appears to be a key motive for 32.9% of patients. Social well-being is also a motivating factor as they want look good when they run into people they don't know (56.6%) and make better first impression in social events (38.4%). More than one-quarter (26.8%) of the cosmetic candidates declare that procedures will allow them stay competitive in their professional field [2]. Increase in popularity of cosmetic medicine can also be attributed to their publicity evoked by celebrities who undergo certain procedures. A prime example of this is Kylie Jenner's announcement in May 2015 that she underwent lip augmentation. Immediately, there was a peak in the popularity of this minimally invasive procedure, as shown by the number of searches via Google search engine. Apart from online searches, lip augmentation procedures performed also increased at that time. Interestingly, its popularity has been sustained in the long term [3].

Another well-known example of celebrity influence on cosmetic procedure volumes is Angelina Jolie's prophylactic mastectomy announcement in *The New York Times* in May 2013. There was massive media coverage that resulted in increased rates of BRCA1 and BRCA2 gene testing and risk-reducing prophylactic mastectomy around the period of Jolie's announcement and the years following. This is now termed as the "Angelina Jolie effect" [3].

Two additional members of the Kardashian family apart from Kylie Jenner who have largely influenced public opinion about cosmetic procedures are Caitlyn Jenner and Kim Kardashian. The first made an announcement in April 2017 about her gender-affirming surgery, and the latter was rumored for her buttock implants in February 2014.

Celebrities may have huge effects on general population engagement in health care, and cosmetic patients who are influenced by them often present in office with their photographs requesting similar changes. This may be an alarming sign during the consultation because it may represent concealed unrealistic expectations. Postoperatively, they may not look like their idols, and this will possibly dissatisfy them.

Thus, the motive for an elective cosmetic procedure may be the desire to look better either for themselves or for others, improving their social status, or following trends set by influencing posts of celebrities. Or maybe they have had a burning desire to correct a flaw in appearance. However, even though many people may have flaws on their appearance, only a portion of them are interested in seeking cosmetic surgery or minimally invasive procedures to fix them.

The great popularity of aesthetic medicine highlights the necessity to identify the psychosocial characteristics of people who are interested in undergoing cosmetic procedures. When physicians are cognitive about their patients' profiles and motivations, they can identify more easily the ones who will benefit from the procedures.

By building a better patient-doctor communication, cosmetic practitioners also benefit themselves from reduced complaints and postsurgery lawsuits [4]. Greater understanding of cosmetic patients may enhance service quality and reduce dissatisfaction. Their motivation, the desires, and needs are valuable clinical information for cosmetic practitioners.

3.2   Motivation for Cosmetic Procedures

As the demand for cosmetic procedures constantly increases, there is need to investigate the factors that create such interest. Motivation to seek a cosmetic procedure is influenced by internal and external factors. The subjective perception and the high or low standards of beauty along with external effect from someone's social network create the desire to alter their appearance.

People perceive beauty in a different way, and this may influence their motivation to seek a cosmetic procedure. Some individuals set high standards when they evaluate beauty and some others not. The concept of aestheticality refers to how people assess human appearance. Aestheticality can be explained by considering a series of 20 pictures—the first a monkey and the last a beautiful woman, with each picture slightly different to its predecessor so that, over the 20 pictures, the metamorphosis is complete. Individuals' choice of where, in the series of pictures, "monkey" ends and "human" begins gives an indication of their "aestheticality." Those with a low level of aestheticality will accept various monkey faces as looking human, and those with a high sense of aestheticality will not accept "human" until all traces of monkey have disappeared. The latter are more prone to be interested in cosmetic procedures [5].

The earliest episode that motivates someone to alter a flaw of their appearance is called sensitization. This may be intrinsic or extrinsic. The first one refers to self-induced thoughts when a child or adolescent looks at themselves at a mirror. Extrinsic sensitization is the result of extraneous remarks or teasing [5].

Extrinsic remarks are significant for the way we evaluate ourselves. At first, parents and relatives express their impressions about a baby's appearance. Self-esteem is considered to be established at that time. Later, children belong to groups that further sensitize them about how they look. Bullying about someone's appearance creates the desire of the bullied child to undergo a cosmetic procedure [6].

Patients sensitized about a feature on their appearance will scrutinize this feature on everyone else—commonly comparing and contrasting. Peer group comparison is common among pupils who are worried about their appearance. They look for a nose/ears/breasts/body which are better, the same, or worse than theirs. Thus, sensitized individuals may express their worries as constant comparison with others and possibly bullying behaviors. This attitude is supported by the image-centered social media. Users encounter dozens of stimuli which may sensitize them to alter their appearance.

During the preoperative consultation, these patients may also scrutinize their appearance to their physician's. Expressions like "your skin is so brighter than mine" or "I wish I had your nose" are repetition of their common habit to make comparisons to other people's characteristics. This behavior may conceal their unrealistic expectations about the cosmetic outcome and should be further investigated.

Table 3.1 Positive predictor of interest in cosmetic surgery

Epidemiologic factors	Female gender
	Low education
Social networks	Knowing someone who has undergone CS
	Teasing history
	Bad relations with parents
	Single marital status
	Having children
Psychological traits	Low body image evaluation
	Dissatisfaction with a specific characteristic
	High body image orientation
	Poor quality of life
	High self-monitoring
	Conscientiousness, agreeability, openness, neuroticism
Psychiatric conditions	Body dysmorphic disorder
	Burnout syndrome
	Narcissistic personality disorder
	Histrionic personality disorder

3.2.1 Predicting Factors of Interest in Cosmetic Procedures

Social acceptance of cosmetic procedures has led to their increased popularity. People want to look younger and fresher and seek either surgical or minimally invasive procedures to achieve that. However, not everyone is equally interested in cosmetic medicine. There are certain psychosocial characteristics that enhance someone's interest in aesthetic procedures [7]. These are categorized in epidemiologic factors, social network characteristics, psychological parameters, and psychopathology (Table 3.1).

3.3 Epidemiologic Factors

3.3.1 Gender

One's physical attractiveness affects the way a person is perceived and treated by others. In modern society, women experience considerable pressure to look young and attractive. One potential consequence would be that women are much more likely to express interest in and receive cosmetic surgery. This explains the ASPS Statistics Report [1] that 92% of cosmetic procedures are performed in women. The total amount of procedures is 14.7 million which includes 1.5 million surgical and 13.3 million minimally invasive procedures.

Frederick et al. analyzed data from 25,714 men and 26,963 women and found that half of the women (48%) were interested in one or more cosmetic procedures, while one-fourth (23%) of men reported such interest ($p < 0.001$) [8]. Consistent with the idea that women are under greater pressure than men to attain current ideals of beauty and thinness, more women than men expressed an interest in cosmetic procedures. The 2018 top five female surgical procedures in the USA have been breast augmentation, liposuction, eyelid surgery, nose reshaping, and abdomino-plasty, and the respective minimally invasive procedures are botulinum toxin type A injections, soft tissue fillers, chemical peel, laser hair removal, and microdermabra-sion [1].

The respective top five surgical list of men includes nose reshaping, eyelid sur-gery, liposuction, breast reduction, and hair transplantation. The top five cosmetic minimally invasive procedures in men are botulinum toxin type A, laser hair removal, microdermabrasion, chemical peels, and soft tissue fillers [1]. Even though men comprise only 8% of cosmetic patients in the USA, the total amount of proce-dures is 1.3 million. Therefore, a substantial minority of men also express some interest and undergo aesthetic procedures suggesting that their perception of beauty, body image, and role in modern societies are evolving. Although women typically outnumber men by an 8:1 ratio among actual cosmetic surgery patients, women in this study [8] outnumbered men by only 2:1 in their interest in cosmetic surgery. Therefore, there are some unknown factors that inhibit men from actually pursuing cosmetic surgery.

3.3.2 Age

The majority of cosmetic procedures are performed in the age group from 40 to 43 years (49% of the total) [1]. People tend to seek procedures to regain their youth. Older women may experience added pressure to obtain rejuvenating procedures because they may feel they are competing with younger women for the attention of their current or potential romantic partners [8]. Age group 13–19 years represent only 1% of the total cosmetic procedures performed, 20–29 years represent 9%, 30–39 years represent 18%, and over 55 years represent 26% of the total number of procedures [1].

Despite this report, there are no clinical studies that consider age as a predictor of the general interest in cosmetic surgery [7]. This may be attributed to the fact that age groups differ regarding the procedures they are interested in. The most popular surgeries of each age group are nose reshaping [13–19], breast augmentation (20–39), liposuction (40–54), and blepharoplasty (55–). Cosmetic patients of vari-ous age groups differ in relation to their specific desires. Therefore, age is not a predictor of general interest of cosmetic procedures.

3.3.3 Body Mass Index (BMI)

BMI is a value derived from the body mass and height of a person. It comprises a convenient rule of thumb to categorize an individual as underweight, normal weight, overweight, or obese based on weight and height. BMI is an independent predictor in certain cosmetic procedures, as in liposuction, regarding both men and women

[9]. That can be interpreted as the false perception of people that liposuction is a weight-losing procedure. In fact, liposuction aims to manage local deposition of fat.

On the contrary, women who decided to undergo breast augmentation mammoplasty are thinner than the general population [10]. This is consistent with current beauty standards of slim and muscular woman with large breasts.

Despite these specific considerations, BMI does not correlate with the general interest in plastic surgery [7]. This can be explained by the diversity of BMI among people who are interested in specific procedures.

3.3.4   Alcohol and Smoking

Smoking and alcohol consumption are common habits that have to be investigated by cosmetic patients. Smoking is an independent factor for negative surgical outcome, causing healing issues and systematic complications. On the other hand, alcohol abuse may conceal impulsivity personality characteristics and more serious psychological problems. In medical literature, they do not seem to correlate with general interest in cosmetic procedures. In specific, alcohol consumption is a predicting factor for interest in breast augmentation [10].

3.3.5   Level of Education

In general, education is related to better health and self-esteem. Even though women with higher education actually have a better opportunity to purchase cosmetic surgery, education seems to be a strong negative predictor of interest in it (OR = 0.58) [9]. Findings of another study also demonstrate that breast augmentation candidates had significantly fewer years of education than controls did [11].

3.4   Social Networks

Social acceptance is a key contributor of the popularity of cosmetic medicine. People generally approve of someone's desire to improve their appearance. This is further supported by sociocultural influence such as mass media over-presentation of beauty standards and cosmetic techniques. Someone's closest social environment like family and friends may also influence their interest in cosmetic medicine.

The average CS candidates exhibit a higher perception of other's opinion [12]. This makes them prone to be vulnerable to seek aesthetic procedures as a result of their social networks.

Knowing someone who has undergone cosmetic surgery is a well-known contributor for interest in cosmetic surgery (OR = 2.89; $p < 0.01$) [13]. People who belong to a social environment that is familiar with aesthetic procedures are nearly three times more likely to seek such procedures themselves. This underlines the fact that people's cosmetic-related behavior is strongly affected by their acquaintance.

School is also a social network which affects children's health-related thoughts and behaviors. People who have been teased for their appearance during childhood and adolescence have a tendency in seeking cosmetic surgery [13, 14]. This relationship is well documented, even though the impact of teasing adults about their appearance is less clear. No association has been found between peer teasing between adults and the likelihood to undergo CS [12]. Therefore, children and adolescents develop long-term interest to alter their appearance following bullying in school. These developmental impacts on body image should further make teachers aware against bullying.

Family is the first and maybe the most important social network for someone's psychosexual development. Psychoanalytic theories suggest that parental unconditional love and support promote children's emotional maturity. Individuals who had been constantly criticized by their parents may have lower self-esteem and occasionally a disturbed body image. Regarding interest in cosmetic surgery, high quality of relationship with parents is a negative predictor (odds ratio [OR = 0.94]; $p = 0.018$) [9].

Marital status is also a significant factor, as fewer women willing to undergo cosmetic surgery were married compared to those not wishing to undergo surgery (odds ratio [OR = 0.47]; $p < 0.01$) [13]. This can be attributed to the feeling of security a life partner may provide or the fact that married women are on average less motivated to enhance their appearance because they do not obtain social or material advantages through this behavior.

On the contrary, having children alters female body and may increase their tendency to seek aesthetic procedures. In medical literature, having children is described as a predictor of interest in cosmetic surgery (odds ratio [OR = 1.70]; $p < 0.001$) [9].

Women's interpersonal relationships and sex-related behaviors are also predictors of interest in breast augmentation mammoplasty. These women have had a greater lifetime number of sexual partners (prevalence odds ratio [pOR] = 8.9), were younger at first pregnancy (pOR = 1.6), are more likely to have a history of terminated pregnancies (pOR = 2.0), and are likely to use oral contraceptives (pOR = 2.2) [10].

3.5   Psychological Traits and Quality of Life

The idea that cosmetic patients are merely motivated either by psychopathology or vanity is outdated. Yet, recent data show that more complex factors including impairment in emotional, social, and professional quality of life may play an important role. The way that people assess their appearance along with their personality characteristics influences their decision to seek cosmetic procedures.

3.5.1 Body Image

Individuals assess their own appearance with different criteria. Some are able to see the objective image, while some others have a disturbed perception of what they look like. These psychological processes consisting of body image and self-esteem are considered key to the motivation for CS. In addition to the objective physical criteria, a number of psychological influences for CS were identified including developmental and sociocultural influences (Table 3.2).

Developmental influences modify children and adolescents in the way they evaluate themselves. Family and peer comments play an important role in the development of their body image. Adults are also affected by numerous sociocultural stimuli like mass media promotion of beauty standards and their interference with emotional and professional success. These processes develop someone's overall body image and satisfaction with specific body parts.

It is not uncommon that cosmetic patients may complain about a specific characteristic of their appearance. Body area dissatisfaction is a strong predictor of interest in CS, and someone's motivation to alter a specific feature of their appearance correlates with their dissatisfaction with this specific characteristic [15]. However, the overall body image is a separate psychological entity. It is comprised of a perceptual and an attitudinal dimension.

Perceptual body image is the dimension that refers to how accurately individuals evaluate their body, whereas the attitudinal dimension relates to individuals' beliefs and feelings about their physical appearance. Attitudinal body image can be further divided into two components, orientation and evaluation (Table 3.3) [16].

Medical literature suggests that investment in daily image-related self-care habits is a predictor of interest in cosmetic surgery. Women who tend to seek aesthetic procedures show higher body image orientation [13, 17, 18]. In fact, people who are motivated to undergo CS have lower global body image evaluation [13] and higher body image orientation [8]. Therefore, they tend to invest more time and money to improve their image and prevent aging.

Table 3.2 Factors that influence body image development

Developmental influence	It refers to childhood and adolescent experiences
Sociocultural influence	It refers to the interaction and effect that social and cultural standards and mass media portrayal of beauty have on the person

Table 3.3 Attitudinal dimension of body image

Body image orientation	Refers to the degree of importance the individuals place on their appearance
Body image evaluation	Refers to how satisfied they are with their body

3.5.2   Self-Esteem

Self-esteem is defined as the evaluation of self-worth and overall feeling about one-self. There is just one study that suggests that when self-esteem declines, male patients seek surgical aesthetic procedures [19]. Additionally, a study of breast augmentation patients recognized self-esteem as a motivating factor for surgery [20]. It may seem logical that people with low self-esteem seek cosmetic changes to augment their moral. Yet, more recent data show that this idea seems outdated. Low self-esteem is not associated with someone's general interest to undergo cosmetic surgery [7]. Instead, cosmetic surgery has a positive effect in patients who undergo a procedure.

3.5.3   Personality Traits

Personality characteristic are stable and independent predictors of health-related habits and attitudes. The top five characteristics are agreeability, extraversion, conscientiousness, neuroticism, and openness. All except for extraversion are associated with someone's higher desire to undergo a cosmetic procedure [9]. Agreeable individuals value getting along with others. They are friendly, trustworthy, and generous. Conscientiousness is the tendency to display self-discipline, stubbornness, and focus on their goals. People with high openness are open to emotion, sensitive to beauty, and willing to try new things. Neuroticism is the tendency to experience negative emotions, such as anger, anxiety, or depression.

Another personality characteristic that plays an important role in someone's interest in seeking cosmetic procedures is self-monitoring. It indicates someone's ability to regulate their behavior in accordance to specific social situations, in other words to monitor their self-presentations. High self-monitorers are persons whose actions are dependent on situational cues, whereas low monitorers' behavior depends more on their inner attitudes and emotion. Higher self-monitoring is associated with someone's greater chance to seek cosmetic procedures [13]. The effect of self-monitoring on the decision to undergo surgery is partially mediated by social acceptance of cosmetic surgery, as high self-monitorers are more aware of the cues indicating social acceptance of CS.

3.5.4   Health-Related Quality of Life

Health-related quality of life (HRQoL) is an individual's perceived physical and mental health over time. There are implications that cosmetic patients report worse HRQoL. The health status of breast reduction patients before treatment and that of a sample of women in the general population has been found to differ. Breast reduction patients functioned significantly worse on all eight dimensions of the SF-36 questionnaire. Of particular note is the difference in the pain score [21]. This suggests that their medical complaint has substantial physical as well as psychosocial components. Abdominoplasty patients reported significantly worse health on five dimensions including role functioning due to physical problems, social function, energy, and the two dimensions measuring psychological functioning and mental health scores, and rhinoplasty patients had significantly lower health perception scores [22]. Cosmetic rhinoplasty patients also reported lower mental health scores, while breast reconstruction patients did not differ significantly from the general population on any SF-36 dimension.

Patients seeking various cosmetic surgical procedures seem to present impaired physical and psychological quality of life. Therefore, cosmetic surgery may function for them as hope to improve it.

3.6   Psychopathology

Cosmetic patients have been commonly accused to be psychologically unstable. Even though that this general assumption is outdated, there are certain psychiatric entities which are associated with increased interest in aesthetic procedures.

Undoubtedly, the most well-known positive predictor for interest in cosmetic surgery is body dysmorphic disorder (BDD). Its incidence does not exceed 1–2% in the general population, whereas 15% of cosmetic patients suffer from BDD-like symptoms [23]. Patients with BDD are characterized by an excessive concern with a minimal or absent flaw in their appearance. A similarly disturbed perception of appearance is noted among individuals with distorted eating behaviors like anorexia nervosa. These cases are also correlated with a fourfold higher interest in plastic surgery (odds ratio [OR] = 4.09; $p < 0.001$).

Burnout syndrome is caused by chronic exposure to stress in a professional environment. Emotional exhaustion and depersonalization are key elements of this psychiatric entity. Burnout-related symptoms have been found to correlate with increased interest in cosmetic surgery [24], suggesting that burnt-out professionals may have a distorted body image or that cosmetic surgery may function as a way to alleviate their emotional exhaustion and depersonalization.

Personality disorders may also influence someone's motivation for cosmetic surgery. These are long-term patterns of behavior and inner experiences that deviate from the expectations of the culture, causing distress or functional impairment.

Narcissistic personality disorder is defined by someone's grandiosity, need for admiration, and lack of empathy. It can be found in 25% of people seeking cosmetic surgery, especially rejuvenating procedures [25]. It is the grandiose sense of self-importance that motivates them to seek cosmetic procedures to improve their appearance. Additionally, people with histrionic personality disorder are presented with emotional excess and the need to gain the attention of others. The prevalence of this personality disorder among cosmetic patients raises up to 9.7% [26]. These individuals may feel uncomfortable when they are not at the center of attention and commonly use physical appearance to draw attention to themselves.

3.7   Conclusion

There are certain psychosocial characteristics that predict general interest in cosmetic surgery. Epidemiologic factors are female gender and low education. Someone's close social environment also plays an important role. Bad relationship with parents, being unmarried, knowing someone who has undergone cosmetic surgery, and having been teased for appearance during childhood increase motivation for CS. Regarding psychological characteristics, low body image evaluation, dissatisfaction with a specific feature, high body image orientation, poor quality of life, high self-monitoring, conscientiousness, openness, neuroticism, and agreeability are positive predictors of interest. Lastly, psychiatric entities that are associated with cosmetic motivation are body dysmorphic disorder, burnout syndrome, and narcissistic and histrionic personality disorders. A better understanding of cosmetic patients and their motivation may lead to better health-care services and positive outcomes.

References

1. ASPS Statistics 2018. https://www.plasticsurgery.org/documents/News/Statistics/2018/plastic-surgery-statistics-full-report-2018.pdf.
2. Maisel A, Waldman A, Furlan K, Weil A, Sacotte K, Lazaroff JM, Lin K, Aranzaru D, Avram MM, Bell A, Cartee TV, Cazzaniga A, Chapas A, Crispin MK, Croix JA, CM DG, Dover JS, Goldberg DJ, Goldman MP, Green JB, Griffin CL, Haimoviv AD, Hausauer AK, Hernandez SL, Hsu S, Ibrahim O, Jones DH, Kaufman J, Kilmer SL, Lee NY, DH MD, Schlessinger J, Tanzi E, Weiss ET, Weiss RA, Wu D, Poon E, Alam M. Self-reported patient motivations for seeking cosmetic procedures. JAMA Dermatol. 2018;154(10):1167–74.
3. Tijerina JD, Morrison SD, Nolan IT, Parham MJ, Richardson MT, Nazerali R. Celebrity influence affecting public interest in plastic surgery procedures: Google trends analysis. Aesthet Plast Surg. 2019;43(6):1669–80.
4. Cole SA. Reducing malpractice risk through more effective communication. Am J Manag Care. 1997;3:649e53.
5. Blackburn VF, Blackburn AV. Taking a history in aesthetic surgery: SAGA – the surgeon's tool for patient selection. J Plast Reconstr Aesthet Surg. 2008;61(7):723–9.
6. Lee K, Guy A, Dale J, Wolke D. Adolescent desire for cosmetic surgery. Associations with bullying and psychological functioning. Plast Reconstr Surg. 2017;139(5):1109–18.
7. Milothridis P, Pavlidis L, Haidich AB, Panagopoulou E. A systematic review of the factors predicting the interest in cosmetic plastic surgery. Indian J Plast Surg. 2016;49(3):397–402.
8. Frederick DA, Lever J, Peplau LA. Interest in cosmetic surgery and body image: views of men and women across the lifespan. Plast Reconstr Surg. 2007;120:1407–15.
9. Javo IM, Sorlie T. Psychosocial predictors of an interest in cosmetic surgery among Norwegian women: a population-based study. Plast Reconstr Surg. 2009;124:2142–8.
10. Cook LS, Daling JR, Voigt LF, DeHart MP, Malone KE, Stanford JL. Characteristics of women with and without breast augmentation. JAMA. 1997;277:1612–7.
11. Didie ER, Sarwer DB. Factors that influence the decision to undergo cosmetic breast augmentation surgery. J Women's Health.
12. Chen HC, Karri V, Yu RL, Chung KP, Lu YT, Yang MC. Psychological profile of Taiwanese female cosmetic surgery candidates: understanding their motivation for cosmetic surgery. Aesthet Plast Surg. 2010;34(3):340–9.

13. von Soest T, Kvalem IL, Skolleborg KC, Roald HE. Psychosocial factors predicting the motivation to undergo cosmetic surgery. Plast Reconstr Surg. 2006;117:51–62.
14. Sarwer DB, LaRossa D, Bartlett SP, Low DW, Bucky LP, Whitaker LA. Body image concerns of breast augmentation patients. Plast Reconstr Surg. 2003;112:83–90.
15. Sarwer DB, Bartlett SP, Bucky LP, LaRossa D, Low DW, Pertschuk MJ, Wadden TA, Whitaker LA. Bigger is not always better: body image dissatisfaction in breast reduction and breast augmentation patients. Plast Reconstr Surg. 1998;101(7):1956–61. (discussion 1962–1963)
16. Cash TF. Body-image attitudes: evaluation, investment, and affect. Percept Mot Skills. 1998;78:1168–70.
17. Ozgur F, Tuncali D, Gursu KG. Life satisfaction, self- esteem, and body image: a psychological evaluation of aesthetic and reconstructive surgery candidates. Aesth Plast Surg. 1998;22:412–9.
18. Sarwer DB, Wadden TA, Pertschuk MJ, Whitaker LA. The psychology of cosmetic surgery: a review and reconceptualization. Clin PsycholRev. 1998;18:1–22.
19. Edgerton CS, Langman MW. Psychiatric considerations. In: Coutiss EH, editor. Male aesthetic surgery. St. Louis: Mosby; 1982. p. 17–38.
20. Solvi AS, Foss K, von Soest T, Roald HE, Skolleborg KC, Holte A. Motivational factors and psychological processes in cosmetic breast augmentation surgery. J Plast Reconstr Aesthet Surg. 2010;63(4):673–80.
21. Klassen A, Fitzpatrick R, Jenkinson C, Goodacre T. Should breast reduction surgery be rationed? A comparison of the health status of patients before and after treatment: postal questionnaire survey. BMJ. 1996;313(7055):454–7.
22. Klassen A, Jenkinson C, Fitzpatrick R, Goodacre T. Patients' health related quality of life before and after aesthetic surgery. Br J Plast Surg. 1996;49(7):433–8.
23. Malick F, Howard J, Koo J. Understanding the psychology of the cosmetic patients. Dermatol Ther. 2008;21:47–53.
24. Milothridis P, Pavlidis L, Panagopoulou E. Are burnt-out doctors prone to seek cosmetic surgery? A cross-sectional study. Aesthet Plast Surg. 2017;41(6):1447–145.
25. Ishigooka J, Iwao M, Suzuki M, Fukuyama Y, Murasaki M, Miura S. Demographic features of patients seeking cosmetic surgery. Psychiatric Clin Neurosci. 1998;52:283–7.
26. Napoleon A. The presentation of personalities in plastic surgery. Ann Plast Surg. 1993;31:193–208.

Bullying About Someone's Appearance and Interest in Cosmetic Surgery

4

Definitions
Bullying: An imbalanced relationship characterized by intended and repeated aggression.

4.1 Introduction

Popularity of cosmetic surgery increases steadily during the early twenty-first century. Social media and mass media coverage of celebrities who undergo esthetic procedures influences potential patients. Maybe more than adults, teenagers are affected by images of beauty and success. In 2018, 17.7 million cosmetic procedures were performed in the USA. Of those procedures, 227,000 were performed in 13–19-year-olds [1]. In general, 64,994 surgical and 162,000 minimally invasive procedures in this age group represent 4% and 1% of the total cosmetic procedures, respectively. The most commonly performed surgical procedures between the age of 13 and 19 are rhinoplasty, breast augmentation, breast reduction in men, otoplasty, and liposuction (Table 4.1). The respective minimally invasive procedures are laser hair removal, laser skin resurfacing, laser treatment of leg veins, and chemical peels (Table 4.2).

Physical appearance plays an important role in school relationships. Beautiful children are more popular than their unattractive peers. Additionally, they seem to be better adjusted [2] and more intellectually competent [3] than less attractive students. Discrimination between pupils further motivates them to get information and seek cosmetic procedures to enhance their appearance.

© Springer Nature Switzerland AG 2020   33
P. Milothridis, *Cosmetic Patient Selection and Psychosocial Background*,
https://doi.org/10.1007/978-3-030-44725-0_4

Table 4.1 Cosmetic surgical procedures (age 13–19) [1]

Cosmetic surgical procedures	Age 13–182,018 total	Age 13–19% of total procedures	Age 13–19% Change 2018 vs. 2017
Rhinoplasty	30,260	14%	−1%
Augmentation mammoplasty	8636	3%	2%
Otoplasty	6391	28%	−3%
Gynecomastia correction	6330	26%	−8%
Liposuction	4164	2%	7%

Table 4.2 Cosmetic minimally invasive procedures (age 13–19) [1]

Cosmetic minimally invasive procedures	Age 13–182,018 total	Age 13–19% of total procedures	Age 13–19% change 2018 vs. 2017
Laser hair removal	69,416	6%	−1%
Laser skin resurfacing	28,880	5%	0%
Botulinum toxin type A	21,575	0,1%	3%
Laser treatment of leg veins	19,464	9%	−2%
Chemical peels	7207	1%	4%

Judgments of physical attractiveness influence students' perceptions of each other, and additionally they appear to influence the relationship between students and teachers. Teachers ascribe more positive attributions to attractive students than unattractive students [4–6]. Teachers perceive beautiful students as having more social skills, confidence, intelligence, and academic potential than their unattractive counterparts.

Beauty bias in the educational system exists in both sides of the student-teacher relationship. Students in first and sixth grades reported that they would prefer to have attractive teachers, believing that they would learn best if they are taught by one [7]. Similarly, middle and high school students described attractive college professors as better ones [8]. These discriminative patterns highlight the importance that members of the school community pose on beauty.

It is obvious that interpersonal relationships in school are significantly influenced by physical appearance. Beauty bias produces both positive interactions and bullying behaviors. Teasing about someone's appearance includes remarks about their height, weight, skin quality and color, prominent ears, nasal shape, and breast size. These aggressive attitudes and teasing about children's appearance seem to disturb their body image and increase their interest in seeking cosmetic procedures both at that time and later during adulthood [9]. Therefore, possible teasing history of cosmetic patients has to be taken into consideration, as this may enhance their interest to undergo esthetic procedures.

4.2   Physiologic and Sociocultural Component of Beauty Perception

Sociocultural influences modify beauty standards to adults. Typically, a superior physical appearance is perceived as a contributor to professional and emotional success in modern societies. However, research shows that perception of beauty in humans has also a physiologic component, as it goes back in puberty. Infants as young as 3 months prefer to look at attractive rather than unattractive faces [10]. They also play for a longer period of time with attractive rather than unattractive dolls [11]. These findings suggest that preferences for beauty result from inner congenital mechanisms rather than socialization.

Later in life, children evaluate their own physical appearance in the mirror and may start to feel dissatisfied with their overall body image or a specific characteristic. The trigger point of dissatisfaction with someone's appearance is called sensitization.

Sensitization is the earliest episode that motivates them to seek cosmetic surgery. It may be intrinsic or extrinsic. The first one refers to self-induced thoughts when a child or adolescent looks at themselves at a mirror. Extrinsic sensitization is the result of extraneous remarks or teasing [12].

A patient sensitized about a feature on his/her appearance will scrutinize this feature on everyone else—always comparing and contrasting. Peer group comparison is common among pupils who are worried about their appearance. They look for a nose/ears/breasts/body which are better, the same, or worse than theirs. Thus, educational environment is an ideal place for the sensitized individuals to express their worries as constant comparison with others. This can lead either to sadness and feelings of inadequacy or aggressive behavior and bullying.

4.3   The Social Burden of Bullying

Bullying is a significant problem of modern educational environments with multiple consequences. It is defined as an imbalanced relationship characterized by intended and unwanted aggressive behavior by another youth or group of youths, who are not siblings or current dating partners [13]. It involves an observed or perceived power imbalance and is repeated multiple times or is highly likely to be repeated [14, 15]. Power imbalance can be expressed via physical, verbal, and psychological violence.

Bullying behaviors are common, as they are reported by one out of five high school students. Regarding gender, bullying and victimization in adolescence among boys and girls is approximately equal: boys tend to be bullies and bully-victims more often than girls, but there are few sex differences in victimization [16–18].

An involved child or adolescent may be a perpetrator (bully), a victim, or both, also known as "bully-victim." Each role is associated with serious consequences. It can have a wide range of adverse effects on children and adolescents including physical, psychological, social, or educational harm [19, 20]. Peer victimization is a childhood trauma that negatively affects psychological functioning, both concurrently and longitudinally [21]. For victims, the negative effects may be similar to those caused by adult abuse or maltreatment [22]. They are at increased risk for depression, anxiety, sleep difficulties, lower academic achievement, and dropping out of school. They also show increased rates of self-harm, suicidal thoughts, and suicide attempts [21]. Bullies are at increased risk for substance use, academic problems, and experiencing violence later in adolescence and adulthood. Interestingly, "bully-victims" suffer the most serious consequences being at greater risk for mental health and behavioral problems.

There are long-term consequences of childhood bullying victimization to adult health outcomes. Being bullied (occasionally or frequently) is associated with higher levels of psychological distress at age 23 and at age 50, almost 40 years after exposure [21]. Poor mental, physical, and cognitive health outcomes at least 40 years after exposure prove that bullying has lasting effects. When bullying remarks focus on characteristics of physical appearance, it may have impact on body image and interest in cosmetic surgery.

4.4   Bullying and Interest in Cosmetic Surgery

In medical literature, it is well established that teasing about someone's appearance during childhood is related to an increased motivation to undergo surgery in adulthood [23]. The possible pathogenetic mechanisms suggest that developmental influences on body image promote a long-term desire to improve their appearance. In fact, the effect of teasing on motivation for cosmetic surgery diminished when the body image variables were included in the analyses, indicating that teasing history has an effect on cosmetic surgery through its effect on body image.

Peers have a large influence on body image, and approximately 50% of adults seeking cosmetic surgery report a history of teasing about their appearance or bullying during childhood or adolescence [24–26].

The negative correlation between teasing history and body image evaluation indicates the latter is influenced by developmental factors. Being bullied is related to poor psychological functioning, for example, reduced body esteem and self-esteem and increased emotional problems [27].

Interaction with other children is a key factor for psychological maturation regarding the way someone evaluates themselves. Interest in cosmetic surgery is influenced by epidemiologic factors, psychological traits, psychiatric entities, and social networks [9]. The latter involves relationship with parents, marital status, knowing someone who has undergone cosmetic surgery, and teasing history.

Therefore, interpersonal factors, such as peer influences, seem to be a significant determinant of someone's motivation to seek cosmetic procedures [23, 25, 26, 28–31].

Teasing during adolescence is not only associated with increased interest in cosmetic surgery later in life but also concurrently. Involvement in bullying in any role was associated with an increased desire of the teenager for cosmetic surgery [27]. The mechanisms were different for those who bully others and those who are bullied (victims and bully-victims). Bullies want to look better independent of their psychological functioning, whereas being bullied was related to reduced psychological functioning, and that partly mediated the effect between being victimized by peers and desire for cosmetic surgery. Victims had the greatest desire for cosmetic surgery and the most extreme scores [27]. Thus, bullying in adolescence not only creates interest in cosmetic surgery to adults with teasing history but also to underage individuals suggesting that it has both an immediate and long-lasting effect.

Specific role models in bullying are associated with different pathogenetic pathways to the interest in cosmetic surgery. On the one hand, bullies seem to desire cosmetic surgery as a need for status and admiration. On the other hand, for the bullied adolescents, it is partly related to their poor psychological functioning. They seem to have reduced body esteem and self-esteem and increased emotional problems.

Children who are exposed to body image comparisons and adverse comments in the educational system may adapt various avoidance behavior patterns. These are strategies to camouflage or avoid exposure of their feature of complaint. These may include choice of clothing and hairstyles but also avoiding sporting activities and in its extreme form going to school. Parents and teachers have to recognize avoiding patterns, as they usually obscure deeper psychological issues.

Consultation with teenagers who seek cosmetic interventions

- Is there an objective indication for the procedure?
- Are there any avoiding behavioral patterns?
- Does the teenager believe that the cosmetic procedure will improve his/her social status at school?
- What is the quality of communication with parents/teachers?

4.5 Conclusion

During consultations, cosmetic professionals have to investigate the history of teasing about their patients' appearance during childhood. This may have caused body image disturbances. Adolescents who seek for cosmetic interventions are likely to be involved in any role of bullying behaviors. Doctors, parents, and teachers have to clarify their motivations, as they may be derived by their need to cope with these conditions.

References

1. ASPS Statistics 2018. https://www.plasticsurgery.org/documents/News/Statistics/2018/plastic-surgery-statistics-full-report-2018.pdf.
2. Langlois JH, Kalakanis L, Rubenstein AJ, Larson A, Hallam MSM. Maxims or myths of beauty? A meta-analytic and theoretical review. Psychol Bull. 2000;126:390–423.
3. Ritts V, Patterson ML, Tubbs ME. Expectations, impressions, and judgements of physically attractive students: a review. Rev Educational Res. 1992;62:413–26.
4. Kenealy P, Frude N, Shaw W. Influence of children's physical attractiveness on teacher's expectations. J Social Psychol. 1988;128:373–83.
5. Lerner RM, Delaney M, Hess LE, Jovanovic J. Early adolescent physical attractiveness and academic competence. J Early Adolescence. 1990;10:4–20.
6. Ritts V, Patterson ML, Tubbs ME. Expectations, impressions, and judgements of physically attractive students: a review. Rev Educational Res. 1992;62:413–26.
7. Hunsberger B, Cavanagh B. Physical attractiveness and children's expectations of potential teachers. Psychol Women Quart. 1988;25:70–4.
8. Romano ST, Bordieri JE. Physical attractiveness stereotypes and students' perceptions of college professors. Psychol Rep. 1989;64:1099–102.
9. Milothridis P, Pavlidis L, Haidich AB, Panagopoulou E. A systematic review of the factors predicting the interest in cosmetic plastic surgery. Indian J Plast Surg. 2016;49(3):397–402.
10. Langlois JH, Roggman LA, Casey RJ, Ritter JM, Rieser-Danner LA, Jenkins VY. Infant preferences for attractive faces: rudiments of a stereotype. Dev Psychol. 1987;23:363–9.
11. Langlois JH, Roggman LA, Rieser-Danner LA. Infants differential social responses to attractive and unattractive faces. Dev Psychol. 1990;26:153–9.
12. Blackburn VF, Blackburn AV. Taking a history in aesthetic surgery: SAGA – the surgeon's tool for patient selection. J Plast Reconstr Aesthet Surg. 2008;61(7):723–9.
13. Centers for Disease Control and Prevention. Understanding bullying. http://www.cdc.gov/violencepreven-tion/pdf/bullying_factsheet.pdf. Accessed 01 Jan 2020.
14. Wolke D, Sapouna M. Big men feeling small: childhood bullying experience, muscle dysmorphia and other mental health problems in bodybuilders. Psychol Sport Exerc. 2008;9:595–604.
15. Wolke D, Lereya ST, Fisher HL, Lewis G, Zammit S. Bullying in elementary school and psychotic experiences at 18 years: a longitudinal, population-based cohort study. Psychol Med. 2014;44:2199–211.
16. Salmivalli C, Lagerspetz K, Björkqvist K, Österman K, Kaukiainen A. Bullying as a group process: participant roles and their relations to social status within the group. Aggress Behav. 1996;22:1–15.
17. Reulbach U, Ladewig EL, Nixon E, O'Moore M, Williams J, O'Dowd T. Weight, body image and bullying in 9-year-old children. J Paediatr Child Health. 2013;49:E288–93.
18. Nansel TR, Overpeck M, Pilla RS, Ruan WJ, Simons-Morton B, Scheidt P. Bullying behaviors among US youth: prevalence and association with psychosocial adjustment. JAMA. 2001;285:2094–100.
19. Fox CL, Farrow CV. Global and physical self-esteem and body dissatisfaction as mediators of the relationship between weight status and being a victim of bullying. J Adolesc. 2009;32:1287–301.
20. Copeland WE, Bulik CM, Zucker N, Wolke D, Lereya ST, Costello EJ. Does childhood bullying predict eating disorder symptoms? A prospective, longitudinal analysis. Int J Eat Disord. 2015;48:1141–9.
21. Takizawa R, Maughan B, Arseneault L. Adult health out- comes of childhood bullying victimization: evidence from a five-decade longitudinal British birth cohort. Am J Psychiatry. 2014;171:777–84.
22. Lereya ST, Copeland WE, Costello EJ, Wolke D. Adult mental health consequences of peer bullying and maltreatment in childhood: two cohorts in two countries. Lancet Psychiatry. 2015;2:524–31.

23. Von Soest T, Kvalem IL, Skolleborg KC, Roald HE. Psychosocial factors predicting the motivation to undergo cosmetic surgery. Plast Reconstr Surg. 2006;117(1):51–62.
24. Markey CN, Markey PM. Correlates of young women's interest in obtaining cosmetic surgery. Sex Roles. 2009;61:158–66.
25. Javo IM, Sørlie T. Psychosocial predictors of an interest in cosmetic surgery among young Norwegian women: a population-based study. Plast Reconstr Surg. 2009;124:2142–8.
26. Jackson AC, Dowling NA, Honigman RJ, Francis KL, Kalus AM. The experience of teasing in elective cosmetic surgery patients. Behav Med. 2012;38:129–37.
27. Lee K, Guy A, Dale J, Wolke D. Adolescent desire for cosmetic surgery. Plast Reconstr Surg. 2017;139(5):1109–18.
28. Delinsky SS. Cosmetic surgery: a common and accepted form of self-improvement? J Appl Soc Psychol. 2005;35:2012–28.
29. Henderson-King D, Brooks KD. Materialism, sociocultural appearance messages, and paternal attitudes predict college women's attitudes about cosmetic surgery. Psychol Women Q. 2009;33:133–42.
30. Brown A, Furnham A, Glanville L, Swami V. Factors that affect the likelihood of undergoing cosmetic surgery. Aesthet Surg J. 2007;27:501–8.
31. Park LE, Calogero RM, Harwin MJ, DiRaddo AM. Predicting interest in cosmetic surgery: interactive effects of appearance-based rejection sensitivity and negative appearance comments. Body Image. 2009;6:186–93.

Body Dysmorphic Disorder: Why Should
Cosmetic Doctors Identify These
Patients?

5

Abbreviations

BDD   Body dysmorphic disorder
OCD   Obsessive–compulsive disorder
SAD   Social anxiety disorder
SRIs   Serotonin reuptake inhibitors

5.1   Introduction

Body dysmorphic disorder (BDD) is a common mental condition which is commonly encountered by cosmetic doctors and aestheticians. It is defined as an excessive preoccupation with one or more perceived defects or flaws in physical appearance that are not observable or appear slight to others. The former term dysmorphophobia has fallen into dispute probably because ICD-10 has discarded it and subsumed it under that of hypochondriacal disorder. The fifth edition of Diagnostic and Statistical Manual (DSM) of Mental Disorders by the American Psychiatric Association includes BDD under a new section for obsessive-compulsive disorders (OCD) [1].

In general population, there are individuals who are dissatisfied with their overall appearance or a specific characteristic. BDD differs from normal appearance concerns due to its association with significant distress which can lead to severe impairment in social status. Anxiety and impaired affective and social functioning are factors that differentiate BDD from normal concerns about someone's appearance [2]. Patients are unable to see the "bigger picture" at the mirror and tend to be focused on small details [3]. This inability has an impact on their thinking and overall perception causing constant concern and ultimately affects negatively their quality of life [4].

© Springer Nature Switzerland AG 2020   41
P. Milothridis, *Cosmetic Patient Selection and Psychosocial Background*,
https://doi.org/10.1007/978-3-030-44725-0_5

Table 5.1 Criteria of BDD diagnosis

Excessive **preoccupation** with one or more perceived defects or flaws in physical appearance that are not observable or slight to others
Concerns are associated with significant **distress** that leads to **social impairment**
Exclusion of other body image disorders (e.g., anorexia nervosa)

The resulting distress causes impairment in their professional life and interpersonal relationships. They are often unemployed or disadvantaged at work, are socially isolated, and are at high risk of committing suicide especially when they have lost all hope of altering their appearance [5]. These potential harmful consequences highlight the significance of an early diagnosis.

The third criterion to establish the diagnosis of BDD is that this preoccupation is not better accounted for by another mental disorder. For example, dissatisfaction with body shape and size is associated with anorexia nervosa. The diagnostic criteria of BDD are summarized in Table 5.1.

Population-based estimates of the prevalence of BDD have ranged from 1.7% to 2.4% [2, 6]. These patients are strongly convinced that appearance flaws are physical rather than psychological. Therefore, they seek cosmetic rather than psychological or pharmaceutical treatment, and the prevalence of BDD among cosmetic surgery patients is much higher. It has been reported to range from 11% to 24% [7]. Another study reports a prevalence as high as 53% [8]. These enormous numbers underline the strong interaction between cosmetic practitioners and BDD patients.

Regarding different medical specialties, a meta-analysis performed on 33 publications concluded that a higher percentage of BDD patients were observed in the specialty of plastic surgery (15.04%) than in dermatology (12.65%) [9]. This can be attributed to their preference for more invasive procedures and radical changes as a result of their significant distress. Regarding different procedures, De Brito et al. [8] studied the prevalence rates of BDD in abdominoplasty, rhinoplasty, and rhytidectomy patients. Abdominoplasty candidates showed the highest prevalence of BDD symptoms (57%), and rhinoplasty candidates had the lower percentage of severe cases ($p < 0.001$).

All cosmetic professionals must be aware of the likelihood of BDD in their patients, especially women aged 25–40 years, who showed a higher prevalence of BDD in the majority of studies. Unfortunately, their satisfaction with the cosmetic outcome is generally low and often leads to the desire to undergo even more procedures [10]. Occasionally, they become either physically or verbally violent toward their doctors. Patients with severe symptoms should be referred to a mental health professional in order to clarify their suitability for cosmetic interventions.

5.2   Clinical Presentation of BDD

BDD shares some similarities with obsessive-compulsive spectrum disorder such as high levels of perfectionism and preference for symmetry. Cosmetic interventions usually aim for improvement rather than perfection. This is something BDD patients fail to accept.

Another related disorder is social anxiety disorder (SAD) because they both share similar pathologic concern of being negatively evaluated by others [11]. This social impairment usually isolates them, as it causes embarrassment and difficulty in developing closer relationships.

BDD patients often spend many hours in time-consuming rituals such as mirror gazing. Sometimes they adopt safety behaviors to reduce showing of the specific feature. Examples are looking down, not allowing others to see their profile, using their hands to hide their characteristic, and wearing large jewelry as distraction. Cosmetic practitioners have to identify these behavioral patterns during preoperative consultation, as they may raise the suspicion of BDD.

Patients with BDD are more likely to seek a cosmetic physician rather than a mental health professional. Their complaints about physical appearance may vary. Either the patient may feel generally ugly or they may be dissatisfied about specific features. Any part of the body may be the focus of BDD, but complaints typically involve perceived or slight flaws on the face or skin such as a feature being too small or too big or not straight, hair thinning, acne, wrinkles, scars, vascular markings, paleness or redness of the complexion, asymmetry, or lack of proportion. Sometimes the complaints are quite vague. Nose seems to be the most common preoccupation in BDD [12].

5.3   Avoidance of Social Situation and Repetitive Behaviors

Delusionality is one of the most debilitating clinical characteristics. Many patients are completely convinced that their perceived defects are real and that others take special notice of their flaws [13]. This is their primary cause of social impairment.

Like patients with OCDs, individuals with body dysmorphic disorder are also characterized by repetitive behaviors like mirror checking, excessive grooming, and skin picking. They often seek for reassurance and compare their appearance with that of others. Self-inspection is also a common characteristic. All these behaviors are defense mechanisms which aim to provide psychological safety to the patients, in terms of their dysfunctional thinking.

5.4   Measurement of BDD

The 34-item Body Dysmorphic Disorder Examination is a specific questionnaire that measures symptoms of severely negative body image. It is used to classify individuals into those with and without BDD symptoms. The items are grouped into six domains assessing preoccupation and negative self-evaluation of appearance, self-consciousness and embarrassment, excessive importance given to appearance in self-evaluation, avoidance of activities, body camouflaging (use of camouflage strategies involving style of clothing, the wearing of accessories, use of makeup, and changes in body posture in an attempt to hide the perceived defect), and body checking (self-inspection, reassurance seeking, and comparing self to others). The items are rated on a scale ranging from 0 to 6, with 0 indicating the absence of negative body image symptoms in the previous four weeks. Scores of 1 to 6 represent the frequency (number of days) or intensity (mild to severe) of symptoms. Total score ranges from 0 to 168, and a cutoff score greater than or equal to 66 indicates a high degree of dissatisfaction with appearance and is associated with a diagnosis of BDD [14].

Even though self-reported questionnaires are accurate to diagnose BDD, they are time-consuming. This is not always practical in terms of a busy cosmetic practice. Additionally, they are not accepted by all patients, as they may feel that they are screened for a psychiatric disorder.

5.5   Are Cosmetic Doctors Aware of BDD?

BDD patients usually continue to be dissatisfied with the characteristic of their appearance postoperatively. The impact of BDD on the postoperative outcome highlights the necessity of cosmetic doctors to identify its signs and act accordingly. In fact, cosmetic professionals have some degree of awareness of body dysmorphic disorder, and this guides their decision of whether or not to perform a procedure. An interesting finding is that plastic surgeons are more inclined than other groups of cosmetic doctors to always share their suspicion of body dysmorphic disorder with their patients. Plastic surgeons also refer more commonly a suspected case to a psychiatrist or psychologist [15].

However, it is not uncommon that patients conceal the nature of the desire to undergo any type of cosmetic procedure. Seeing over 500 candidate cosmetic patients per year, 83.2% of the professionals recognized between one and ten BDD patients, which is lower (i.e., maximum 2%) than would be expected given the 10% prevalence of BDD in these settings [15]. The findings of Sarwer [16] and Szepietowski et al. [17] carry a similar impression that might be interpreted as underdiagnosis. On the contrary, dermatologists identified approximately 13% of BDD patients in their practice, a significantly higher percentage probably lying close to reality.

5.6   Consequences of BDD

The clinical significance of identification of these patients lies in the poor postoperative outcome following cosmetic procedures. Additionally, BDD is associated with poor quality of life and risky behaviors. Patients with BDD are susceptible to self-destructive behaviors. High suicidal ideation (80%) and suicide attempt (24%) rates are found among them [18]. Suicide rate among individuals with BDD is 45 times higher than that in the general US population, with a mortality rate higher than those with anorexia nervosa, major depression, and bipolar disorder. Their impulsivity may lead to aggressiveness, eating disorders, repeated hospitalizations, and obsessive desire to undergo cosmetic procedures.

They also tend to be linked to extreme behaviors such as "do-it-yourself" (DIY) cosmetic surgery in an attempt to correct the perceived defect. History of DIY cosmetic procedures is an alarming sign during preoperative consultation.

5.7   Treatment of BDD

When there is suspicion of BDD, cosmetic doctors should refer patients for evaluation by a mental health professional. In fact, most patients feel ashamed to seek treatment by a psychiatrist or psychologist, and it is very likely that they do not agree with the referral. However, they significantly benefit from psychotherapy and pharmaceutical treatment.

Pharmaceutical options include the SRIs like fluoxetine, fluvoxamine, citalopram, escitalopram, and clomipramine [19]. They improve BDD symptoms in 53% to 73% of the patients. The mean response time is 4 to 9 weeks. SRIs seem to be efficacious even for delusional BDD patients. Medication should be given long term because discontinuation seems to increase relapse rate [20].

Nonpharmacologic treatment options include cognitive behavioral therapy (CBT). A typical course of CBT for BDD involves 18 to 22 sessions with several core treatments such as psychoeducation, motivational enhancement, cognitive restructuring, in vivo exposures and response prevention, perceptual mirror retraining, and relapse prevention [21]. Cognitive technique mainly focuses on knowing the factors that have contributed to the development of BDD, evaluating the accuracy of maladaptive thoughts, and working toward developing more adaptive beliefs. Behavioral therapy includes techniques of exposure to situations that make patient nervous and response prevention. For example, during mirror checking patients are trained to describe themselves in an objective, nonjudgmental manner while standing at least an arm away from the mirror. This allows for the anxiety to subside but also promotes more objective ways of describing appearance in consistency to cognitive therapy and disrupts the typical manner in which patients relate to the mirror.

Psychiatric treatment seems to be the optimal treatment for these patients. Retrospective studies of BDD patients attending psychiatric clinics suggest a poor outcome following cosmetic surgery, so it is generally not recommended for them. A randomized controlled study would have more objective conclusion, but such trial would raise ethical concerns [22].

Even though BBD has been traditionally considered to be a contraindication for aesthetic surgery, more recent data show that patients with mild to moderate symptoms may benefit from cosmetic procedures [23]. This is further supported by another study which showed that there is a group of patients with subclinical or very mild BDD who are satisfied by cosmetic rhinoplasty [22].

Nevertheless, cosmetic professionals need to identify BDD during preoperative consultation. Most of the professionals take their time to address body image problems and incorporate psychological consultation or care into their approach. They have some degree of awareness, and this guides their decision of whether or not to perform a decision [24].

5.8   Clinical Tool to Identify Possible BDD Patients

Even though cosmetic doctors are generally aware of the possible presence of BDD in their clinical practice, their task to identify these patients is difficult. There is lack of evidenced-based clinical tools, and also some patients are able to conceal their condition. An algorithm regarding identification of BDD to help cosmetic professionals during patient selection is presented (Fig. 5.1).

During preoperative consultation, cosmetic physicians have to evaluate the objective degree of the perceived flaw of the appearance. If this is presented greater than it is in reality, then the first suspicion of BDD is produced. Cosmetic professionals are suggested not to undervalue immediately the degree of deformity, so as to further investigate their patients' condition.

Secondly, they should investigate the level of distress that patients may feel about the perceived flaw in their appearance. This is evaluated primarily by the way that patients talk about their problem. Loud speaking and exaggerated words of distress

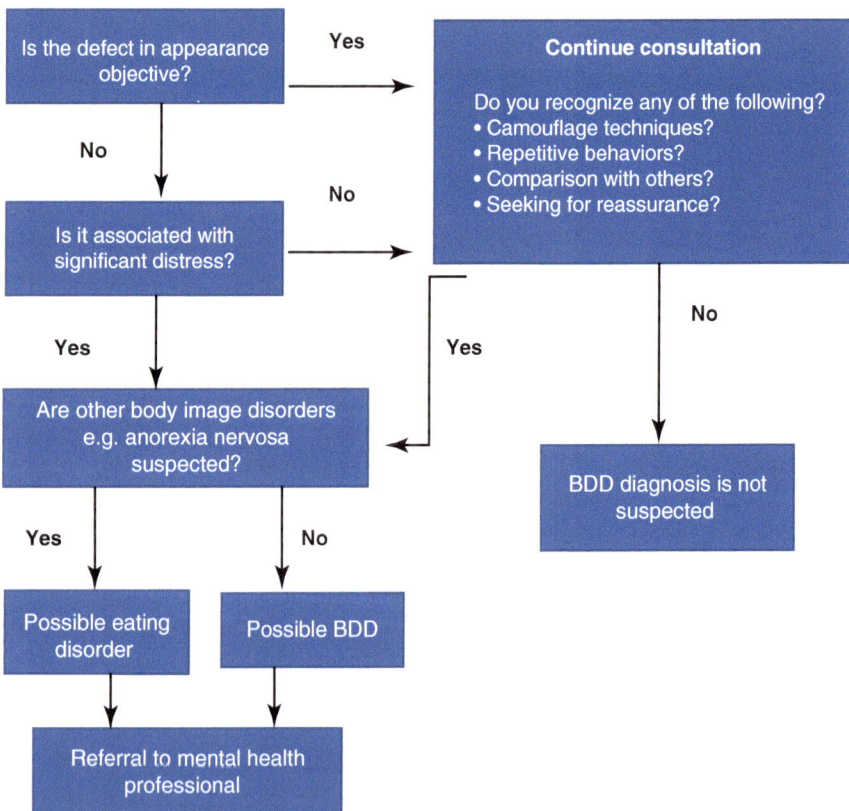

Fig. 5.1 An algorithm to identify BDD patients during preoperative consultation

are suspicious marks. Impairment of their social life because of their appearance has to be excluded. Physician may also make the following questions:

- Do you think about your deformity multiple times during the day?
- Is it an important problem for you?
- Do you feel like you are unlucky because of your appearance?
- Do you think that your appearance is a drawback for your career/relationships?
- Do you believe that people note this feature when they first meet you?
- Would your career be better if you alter this feature?

In cases that the above signs are positive, cosmetic professionals have to exclude other body image disorders like anorexia nervosa. Body mass index (BMI) less than 17.5 should raise the suspicion for the presence of an eating disorder. Unwillingness to calculate someone's weight is also a suspicious sign.

Even if all of the three abovementioned criteria are positive, the cosmetic physician has to continue the preoperative in order to obtain a complete report of the patient. During the visit, the following alarming signs are also noted.

- Techniques to camouflage the defect. Excessive makeup; proper garment and accessories, e.g., large earrings; and avoidance to show the characteristic or their profile are the first alarming signs. BDD patients may also use their hand to cover the characteristic during the interaction with the doctor.
- Repetitive behaviors. Patients who grab a handheld mirror and constantly look at themselves represent individuals at high risk for BDD diagnosis. They use mirrors in an attempt to display the characteristic that they are worried about, simply because it is not obvious enough. Constant self-inspection is an alarming sign of BDD.
- Constantly touching the characteristic trying to improve it temporarily.
- Aggressively picking their skin.
- History of "do-it-yourself" procedures at home. Patients rarely admit having done them, but the physician can identify their possible complications. Application of deep peels may cause permanent burn scars or hyper- and hypopigmentation, and injectable fillers may produce unnatural results. Patients may even undergo self-surgery under local anesthesia attempting to correct the flaw.
- People who call themselves perfectionists are notorious to be bad candidates. They have to understand preoperatively that the goal of the cosmetic procedure is improvement rather than perfection.
- Candidates who ask for symmetrical results. Desire for an absolute symmetry is a sign of OCD. In fact, human faces are seldom symmetrical.
- Comparing themselves with others, e.g., the physician. BDD patients may admire cosmetic physician's characteristics and typically say that they would like to look like them. Otherwise, they may bring photographs of celebrities or edited images of themselves asking for an identical result.
- Seeking for reassurance. BDD patients commonly seek indirectly for the physician's comments that the characteristic is acceptable.

Empathy is an important clinical ability of cosmetic doctors during preoperative consultation. It can help patients reveal their inner thoughts about their condition.

5.9   Conclusion

Body dysmorphic patients represent a significant proportion of cosmetic candidates. As their postoperative satisfaction is usually compromised and patients may be self-destructive or violent toward their physician, careful screening during preoperative consultation is mandatory. The suggested clinical tool may prove to be useful for cosmetic physicians to identify BDD patients during preoperative visits.

References

1. American Psychiatric Association. Diagnostic and statistical manual of mental disorder. 5th ed. Washington, DC: Author; 2013.
2. Koran LM, Abujaoude E, Large MD, Serpe RT. The prevalence of body dysmorphic disorder in the United States adult population. CNS Spectr. 2008;13:316–22.
3. Feusner JD, Yaryura-Tobias J, Saxena S. The pathophysiology of body dysmorphic disorder. Body Image. 2008;5:3–12.
4. Phillips KA, Didie ER, Feusner J, Wilhelm S. Body dysmorphic disorder: treating an under-recognized disorder. Am J Psychiatry. 2008;165(9):1111–8.
5. Veale D, Boocock A, Gournay K, Dryden W, Shah F, Willson R, Walburn J. Body dysmorphic disorder. A survey of fifty cases. Br J Psychiatry. 1996;169:196–201.
6. Buhlmann U, Glaesmer H, Mewes R, Fama JM, Wilhem S, Brahler E, Rief W. Updates on the prevalence of body dysmorphic disorder: a population-based study. Psychiatry Res. 2010;178(1):171–5.
7. Bellino S, Zizza M, Paradiso E, Rivarossa A, Fulcheri M, Bogetto F. Dysmorphic concern symptoms and personality disorders: a clinical investigation in patients seeking cosmetic surgery. Psychiatry Res. 2006;144(1):73–8.
8. De Brito MJ, Nahas FX, Cordas TA, Tavares H, Ferreira LM. Body Dysmorphic disorder in patients seeking abdominoplasty, and rhytidectomy. Plast Reconstr Surg. 2016;137(2):462–71.
9. Ribeiro RVE. Prevalence of body Dysmorphic disorder in plastic surgery and dermatology patients: a systematic review with meta-analysis. Aesthet Plast Surg. 2017;41(4):964–70.
10. Phillips KA, Grant J, Siniscalchi J, Albertini RS. Surgical and nonpsychiatric medical treatment of patients with body dysmorphic disorder. Psychosomatics. 2001;42:504–10.
11. Coles ME, Phillips KA, Menard W, et al. Body dysmorphic disorder and social phobia: cross-sectional and prospective data. Depress Anxiety. 2006;23:26–33.
12. Phillips KA, McElroy SL, Keck PE Jr, Pope HG Jr, Hudson JI. Body dysmorphic disorder: 30 cases of imagined ugliness. Am J Psychiatry. 1993;150:302–8.
13. Eisen JL, Phillips KA, Coles ME, et al. Insight in obsessive compulsive disorder and body dysmorphic disorder. Compr Psychiatry. 2004;45:10–5.
14. Phillips KA. Body image and body dysmorphic disorder. In: Cash TF, Pruzinsky T, editors. Body image: a handbook of theory, research, and clinical practice, vol. 36. New York: the Guilford Press; 2004. p. 312–22.
15. Bouman TK, Mulkens S, van der Lei B. Cosmetic professionals' awareness of body Dysmorphic disorder. Plast Reconstr Surg. 2017;139(2):336–42.
16. Sarwer DB. Awareness and identification of body dysmorphic disorder by aesthetic surgeons: results of a survey of American Society for Aesthetic Plastic Surgery members. Aesthet Surg J. 2002;22:531–5.

17. Szepietowski JC, Salomon J, Pacan P, Hrehorów E, Zalewska A. Body dysmorphic disorder and dermatologists. J Eur Acad Dermatol Venereol. 2008;22:795–9.
18. Phillips KA. Suicidality in body dysmorphic disorder. Prim Psychiatry. 2007;14(12):58–66.
19. Fang A, Matheny NL, Wilhelm S. Body dysmorphic disorder. Psychiatr Clin N Am. 2014;37(3):287–300.
20. Phillips KA, Albertini RS, Siniscalchi JM, Khan A, Robinson M. Effectiveness of pharmacotherapy for body dysmorphic disorder: a chart-review study. J Clin Psychiatry. 2001;62:721–7.
21. Veale D. Cognitive behavioral therapy for body dysmorphic disorder. Psychiatric Ann. 2010;40:333–40.
22. Veale D, De Haro L, Lambrou C. Cosmetic rhinoplasty in body dysmorphic disorder. Br J Plast Surg. 2003;56(6):546–51.
23. Felix GA, de Brito MJ, Nahas FX, Tavares H, Cordas TA, Dini GM, Ferreira LM. Patients with mild to moderate body dysmorphic disorder may benefit from rhinoplasty. J Plast Reconstr Aesthet Surg. 2014;67:646–54.
24. Bouman TK, Mulkens S, van der Lei B. Cosmetic professionals' awareness of body dysmorphic disorder. Plas Reconstr Surg. 2017;139(2):336–42.

Do Psychiatric Disorders Influence Interest in Cosmetic Procedures?

6.1   Introduction

Research conducted between the 1950s and 1970s indicated that a majority of cosmetic surgery patients suffered from psychopathology [1]. Most of these studies relied on clinical interviews of patients conducted by psychoanalytically trained psychiatrists [2]. The most common diagnoses of cosmetic candidates were personality disorders, with smaller percentages of them being characterized as neurotic or psychotic.

In a study of 72 surgical rejuvenating cases from 1965 [3], differences were noted regarding patient age. The 29- to 39-year-old group had more childish behavior, more difficulty in considering parental roles, and more strained relationships with their own parents. The 40- to 50-year-olds were intensely committed to their professional life and sought occupational advantages from a more youthful appearance. They also gave less priority to their personal relationships. In the over 50 group, 90% had lost close relatives within 5 years, and many showed symptoms of unresolved grief reactions. Some believed that surgery will alleviate their sadness.

Gillies [4] suggested that men presenting for rhinoplasty are expressing a prodromal symptom of schizophrenia (monosymptomatic hypochondriacal psychosis), and Gibson [5] and Edgerton [6] also supported this. These abnormal findings quickly became a common belief among general population. At that time, there were some social clichés about aesthetic medicine. The stereotypical cosmetic patients were thought to be a wealthy, neurotic, and narcissist individuals who were constantly trying to polish their exteriors, because they lacked an interesting personality.

During the 1970s, other interview research also found high rates of psychopathology. Prospective patients in several studies were described as experiencing increased symptoms of depression and anxiety, as well as low self-esteem. Although these interview studies have been consistent in their outcomes, they typically suffered from significant methodological problems. The majority of them lacked uniform diagnostic criteria and comparison groups. The latter makes it impossible to

© Springer Nature Switzerland AG 2020
P. Milothridis, *Cosmetic Patient Selection and Psychosocial Background*,
https://doi.org/10.1007/978-3-030-44725-0_6

determine if the reported level of psychological distress is greater than that of general population or other medical patients [7].

In contrast, later studies that used valid psychometric measures have found less psychopathology among cosmetic patients. Either their characteristics have changed over time or the earlier studies had serious methodological drawbacks, yet the findings that the majority of cosmetic patients have little psychopathology are more consistent with the experiences of present cosmetic physician.

Therefore, the idea that psychopathology is very common among cosmetic patients is outdated [8, 9]. During the 1960s, there seemed to be a lower threshold than today to ascertain whether a patient suffered from a psychiatric disease [10]. Nevertheless, cosmetic doctors notice that their patients have certain psychosocial characteristics. Epidemiologic factors, social networks, personality traits, and psychopathology predict interest in aesthetic procedures. Psychological disorders are more common in patients seeking cosmetic surgery than in general population [11, 12].

Prevalence of past or current psychiatric symptoms among US elective cosmetic patient seems to be as high as 44.1% [13]. Like the US general population, depression and anxiety were found to be the most common diagnoses [14–16]. Sufferers may believe that cosmetic procedures will alleviate their symptoms.

Another well-known example of psychiatric condition is body dysmorphic disorder (BDD). BDD patients perceive a slight or absent defect of their appearance as significant. Thus, they seek for an aesthetic procedure to fix it. Even though they represent 1% of general population, their incidence among cosmetic patients is about 15%. Doctors must exclude BDD during preoperative consultation, as sufferers are rarely satisfied with the result [17–22].

Cosmetic professionals must be aware of any psychiatric medication for past or current conditions of their patients. As some psychiatric entities may predict interest in aesthetic procedures and the postoperative benefit, cosmetic physicians have to investigate their presence and refer these patients to a mental health professional if necessary.

6.2   Are Psychiatric Consultations Common Among Cosmetic Patients?

The Diagnostic and Statistical Manual of Mental Disorders (DSM) is a publication for the classification of mental disorders using a common language and common criteria. The DSM-IV classification is organized in a five-part axial system. The first axis incorporated all clinical disorders. The second axis covered personality disorders and intellectual disabilities.

Even though the idea that people who are interested in cosmetic procedures are mentally instable, there are reports of high psychological morbidity among them. In a study of 415 patients seeking cosmetic surgery, 198 (47.7%) were found to have mental disorders according to ICD-10 including 47 with neurotic disorders, 42 with hypochondriacal disorders, 33 with depressive episode, 20 with persistent delusional disorders, 17 with schizophrenia, and 14 with histrionic personality disorder [23]. The rate of individuals with poor social adjustment was 56%. In this study, male subjects were more likely to have a psychiatric disorder. This supports the idea that male cosmetic candidates are potentially problematic.

6.3   Body Dysmorphic Disorder

Body dysmorphic disorder (BDD) is a mental condition which is commonly encountered by cosmetic doctors and aestheticians. It is defined as an excessive preoccupation with one or more perceived defects or flaws in physical appearance that are not observable or appear slight to others. The former term dysmorphophobia has fallen into dispute probably because ICD-10 has discarded it and subsumed it under that of hypochondriacal disorder. The fifth edition of the Diagnostic and Statistical Manual (DSM) of Mental Disorders by the American Psychiatric Association includes BDD under a new section for obsessive-compulsive disorders (OCD) [24].

In general population, there are also individuals who are dissatisfied with their overall appearance or a specific characteristic. BDD differs from normal appearance concerns due to its association with significant distress which can lead to severe impairment in social status. Anxiety and impaired affective and social functioning are factors that differentiate BDD from normal concerns about someone's appearance [25]. Patients are unable to see the "bigger picture" at the mirror and tend to be focused on small details [26]. This inability has an impact on their thinking and overall perception causing constant concern and ultimately affects negatively their quality of life [27].

The resulting distress causes impairment in their professional life and interpersonal relationships. They are often unemployed or disadvantaged at work, are socially isolated, and are at high risk of committing suicide especially when they have lost all hope of altering their appearance [28].

The third criterion to establish the diagnosis of BDD is that this preoccupation is not better accounted for by another mental disorder. For example, dissatisfaction with body shape and size is associated with anorexia nervosa. The diagnostic criteria of BDD are summarized in Table 6.1.

The potentially harmful consequences of BDD highlight the significance of an early diagnosis. Population-based estimates of the prevalence of BDD have ranged from 1.7% to 2.4% [25, 29]. These patients are strongly convinced that appearance flaws are physical rather than psychological. Therefore, they seek cosmetic rather than psychological or pharmaceutical treatment, and the prevalence of BDD among

Table 6.1   Criteria of BDD diagnosis

Excessive **preoccupation** with one or more perceived defects or flaws in physical appearance that are not observable or slight to others
Concerns are associated with significant **distress** that leads to **social impairment**
Exclusion of other body image disorders (e.g., anorexia nervosa)

cosmetic surgery patients is much higher. It has been reported to range from 11% to 24% [30]. Another study reports a prevalence as high as 53% [31]. These enormous numbers underline the strong interaction between cosmetic practitioners and BDD patients.

6.4   Comorbidity in Cosmetic Surgery-Seeking Patients with BDD

There are additional psychiatric disorders that have been investigated in BDD patients who seek cosmetic surgery [32]. They appear to have high prevalence rates of several comorbid Axis I disorders including major depression, social phobia, and obsessive-compulsive disorder. Compared to patients without BDD seeking cosmetic surgery, those with BDD also have significantly higher rates of Axis II disorders including borderline, avoidant, paranoid, schizotypal, and obsessive-compulsive personality disorders.

6.5   Depression

Depressive disorders can be considered one of the major challenges in medicine in view of their high and steadily increasing incidence and their debilitating consequences. They currently affect over 350 million individuals around the world and are the second cause of disease in terms of disability-adjusted life years in the 15–44-year-old age group for both sexes [33]. It is estimated that in 2020 depressive disorders will be the principal cause of disability in both sexes in any age group in developing countries and the second most common cause in developed countries, following ischemic heart disease. By 2030, depression is thought to be the most common disease worldwide, in any age and sex [34].

There is evidence that the prevalence of depression is greater in cosmetic patients than in general population [16, 35, 36]. It is assumed that in a portion of cosmetic patients, DD is the consequence of dissatisfaction with body image, whereas in others it is the result of inner mechanisms. The first ones may benefit from the procedure in terms of psychological function, but for the latter the unrealistic expectations that cosmetic procedure will solve their problems may prove catastrophic.

Of patients undergoing body-contouring surgery, 45% report of having had an episode of depression during their lifetime and 3.8% having taken antidepressant drug therapy [37]. The incidence of suicide in patients with depression is 30-fold than that of general population. This may be relevant with the finding that women with breast implants have a two to three times increased risk of committing suicide. In fact, the prevalence of depressive symptoms (DS) was found in 18.9% of cosmetic breast surgery patients [38]. Another interesting finding of the study is that patients who are presented in public institutions have a 2.3 times greater risk of having DS than those presented in private institutions. This is useful for cosmetic surgeons working in public hospitals to know.

6.6   Anxiety

Anxiety is an emotion characterized by an unpleasant state of inner turmoil, often accompanied by nervous behavior such as pacing back and forth, somatic complaints, and rumination [39].

It may be expressed in various ways. The physiological symptoms of anxiety may include:

- Neurological, as headache, paresthesias, fasciculations, vertigo, or presyncope.
- Digestive, as abdominal pain, nausea, diarrhea, indigestion, dry mouth, or bolus.
- Respiration, as shortness of breath or sighing breathing.
- Cardiac, as palpitations, tachycardia, or chest pain.
- Muscular, as fatigue, tremors, or tetany.
- Cutaneous, as perspiration or itchy skin.
- Urogenital, as frequent urination, urinary urgency, dyspareunia, impotence, or chronic pelvic pain syndrome. Stress hormones released in an anxious state have an impact on bowel function.

6.7   Social Anxiety Disorder (SAD)

The defining feature of SAD, also called social phobia, is intense anxiety or fear of being judged, negatively evaluated, or rejected in a social performance situation. Humans generally require social acceptance and thus sometimes dread the disapproval of others. Apprehension of being judged by others may cause anxiety in social environments.

Social anxiety has behavioral, cognitive, and affective effects. Individuals may become avoidant, antagonistic, or even hostile. It has multiple consequences, and patients use coping mechanisms, as an attempt to improve their quality of life. If the cause of their anxiety is dissatisfaction with appearance or feelings of embarrassment about a body part, they tend to seek cosmetic procedures to alleviate their symptoms. A study of patients seeking cosmetic surgery found that the rate of individuals with poor social adjustment was 56% [23].

6.8   Personality Disorders

Personality disorders are a class of mental disorders characterized by enduring maladaptive patterns of behavior, cognition, and inner experience, exhibited across many contexts and deviated by the individual's culture. They develop early in someone's life and are associated with significant distress and disability.

A study of cosmetic patients undergoing body-contouring surgery found a prevalence of personality disorders among 32% of the sample [37]. Schizoid type (11.49%), histrionic (9.19%), and borderline (6.18%) personality disorders are among the most common.

6.9   Schizoid Personality Disorder (SPD)

SPD is a personality disorder characterized by a lack of interest in social relationships, a tendency toward solitary or sheltered lifestyles, secretiveness, emotional coldness, detachment, and apathy. Bullying is particularly common toward them, and suicide may be a running mental theme for schizoid individuals, though they are not likely to attempt one. (https://en.wikipedia.org/wiki/Schizoid_personality_disorder).

6.10   Borderline Personality Disorder (BPD)

BPD also known as emotionally unstable personality disorder is characterized by a long-term pattern of unstable relationships, a distorted sense of self, and strong emotional reactions. There are often self-harm and other dangerous behaviors. Substance abuse, depression, and eating disorders are commonly associated with BDP. Up to 10% of people affected die of suicide.

6.11   Histrionic Personality Disorder (HPD)

HPD is defined as a personality disorder characterized by a pattern of excessive attention-seeking emotions, inappropriately seductive behavior, and an excessive need for approval. Histrionic traits are marked by the search of attention, frequently using the physical aspect to attract it. Therefore, interest in cosmetic procedures is attributed by the desire for attention and approval from society, rather for internal satisfaction.

6.12   Narcissistic Personality Disorder (NPD)

NPD is a personality characterized by a long-term pattern of exaggerated feelings of self-importance, an excessive need for admiration, and a lack of empathy toward other people. They often spend much time thinking about achieving power and success. As a result of these characteristics, they tend to seek cosmetic procedures to achieve an impressive appearance.

6.13   Conclusion

Various psychiatric disorders are associated with an increased interest in cosmetic procedures. Among them, BDD, depression, social anxiety disorder, burnout syndrome, and personality disorders influence someone's cosmetic motivation. Physicians must identify these patients during preoperative consultation and refer them to a mental health professional, as their psychiatric condition may predict a poor postoperative outcome.

References

1. Edgerton MT, Jacobson WE, Meyer E. Surgical-psychiatric study of patients seeking plastic (cosmetic) surgery: 98 consecutive patients with minimal deformity. Br J Plast Surg. 1960;13:136–45.
2. Grossbart TA, Sarwer DB. Psychosocial issues and their relevance to the cosmetic surgery patient. Semin Cutan Med Surg. 2003;22(2):136–47.
3. Webb WL, Slaughter R, Meyer E. Mechanisms of psychosocial adjustments in patients seeking "face-lift" operation. Psychosomatic Med. 1965;27:183–92.
4. Gillies H. Clinical diagnosis of early schizophrenia. In: Roger TF, Mowbray RM, Roy IR, editors. Topics in psychiatry. London: Hodder and Stoughton; 1958.
5. Gipson M, Connolly FH. The incidence of schizophrenia and severe psychological disorders in patients 10 years after cosmetic rhinoplasty. Br J Plast Surg. 1975;28:155.
6. Edgerton MT, Meyer E, Canter A, Slaughter R. Psychiatric evaluation of male patients seeking cosmetic surgery. Plast Reconstr Surg Transplant Bull. 1960;26:356–72.
7. Sarwer DB, Pertschuk MJ, Wadden TA, Whitaker LA. Psychological investigations of cosmetic surgery patients: a look back and a look ahead. Plast Reconstr Surg. 1998;101:1136–42.
8. Wright MR, Wright WK. A psychological study of patients undergoing cosmetic surgery. Arch Otolaryngol. 1975;101:145–51.
9. Ferraro GA, Rossano F, D'Andrea F. Self-perception and self- esteem of patients seeking cosmetic surgery. Aesthet Plast Surg. 2005;29:184–9.
10. Meyer E, Jacobsen WE, Edgerton MT, Canter A. Motivational patterns in patients seeking elective plastic surgery: I. women who seek rhinoplasty. Psychosom Med. 1960;22:193–203.
11. Sarwer DB, Pertschuk MJ, Wadden TA, Whitaker LA. Psychological investigations in cosmetic surgery: a look back and a look ahead. Plast Reconstr Surg. 1998;101:1136–42.
12. Castle DJ. Mental health histories and psychiatric medication us-age among persons who sought cosmetic surgery (discussion). Plast Reconstr Surg. 2004;114:1934.
13. Jang B, Bhavsar DR. The prevalence of psychiatric disorder among elective cosmetic patients. Eplasty. 2019;19:e6.
14. Schlebusch L, Mahrt I. Long-term psychological sequelae of augmentation mammoplasty. S Afr Med J. 1993;83:267–71.
15. Vargel S, Uluşahin A. Psychopathology and body image in cosmetic surgery patients. Aesthet Plast Surg. 2001;25:474–8.
16. Alagöz MS, Başterzi AD, Uysal AC, Tuzer V, Unlu RE, Sensoz O, Goka E. The psychiatric view of patients of aesthetic surgery: self-esteem, body image, and eating attitude. Aesthet Plast Surg. 2003;27:345–8.
17. Sarwer DB, Wadden TA, Pertschuk MJ, Whitaker LA. Body image dissatisfaction and body dysmorphic disorder in 100 cosmetic surgery patients. Plast Reconstr Surg. 1998;101(6):1644–9.
18. Sarwer DB. Awareness and identification of body dysmorphic disorder by aesthetic surgeons: results of a survey of American Society for Aesthetic Plastic Surgery members. Aesthet Surg J. 2002;22(6):531–5.
19. Sarwer DB, Crerand CE, Didie ER. Body dysmorphic disorder in cosmetic surgery patients. Facial Plast Surg. 2003;19(1):7–18.
20. Sarwer DB, Crerand CE. Body dysmorphic disorder and appearance enhancing medical treatments. Body Image. 2008;5(1):50–8.
21. Marques L, Weingarden HM, Leblanc NJ, Wilhelm S. Treatment utilization and barriers to treatment engagement among people with body dysmorphic symptoms. J Psychosom Res. 2011;70(3):286–93.

22. Javanbakht M, Nazari A, Javanbakht A, Moghaddam L. Body dysmorphic factors and mental health problems in people seeking rhinoplastic surgery. Acta Otorhinolaryngol Ital. 2012;32(1):37–40.

23. Ishigooka J, Iwao M, Suzuki M, Fukuyama Y, Murasaki M, Miura S. Demographic features of patients seeking cosmetic surgery. Psychiatry Clin Neurosci. 1998;52:283–7.

24. American Psychiatric Association. Diagnostic and statistical manual of mental disorder. 5th ed. Washington, DC: Author; 2013.

25. Koran LM, Abujaoude E, Large MD, Serpe RT. The prevalence of body dysmorphic disorder in the United States adult population. CNS Spectr. 2008;13:316–22.

26. Feusner JD, Yaryura-Tobias J, Saxena S. The pathophysiology of body dysmorphic disorder. Body Image. 2008;5:3–12.

27. Phillips KA, Didie ER, Feusner J, Wilhelm S. Body dysmorphic disorder: treating an under-recognized disorder. Am J Psychiatry. 2008;165(9):1111–8.

28. Veale D, Boocock A, Gournay K, Dryden W, Shah F, Willson R, Walburn J. Body dysmorphic disorder. A survey of fifty cases. Br J Psychiatry. 1996;169:196–201.

29. Buhlmann U, Glaesmer H, Mewes R, Fama JM, Wilhem S, Brahler E, Rief W. Updates on the prevalence of body dysmorphic disorder: a population-based study. Psychiatry Res. 2010;178(1):171–5.

30. Bellino S, Zizza M, Paradiso E, Rivarossa A, Fulcheri M, Bogetto F. Dysmorphic concern symptoms and personality disorders: a clinical investigation in patients seeking cosmetic surgery. Psychiatry Res. 2006;144(1):73–8.

31. De Brito MJ, Nahas FX, Cordas TA, Tavares H, Ferreira LM. Body dysmorphic disorder in patients seeking abdominoplasty, and rhytidectomy. Plast Reconstr Surg. 2016;137(2):462–71.

32. Sansone R, Sansone L. Cosmetic surgery and psychological issues. Psychiatry. 2007;4(12):65–8.

33. McGrath MH, Mukerji S. Plastic surgery and the teenage patient. J Pediatr Adolesc Gynecol. 2000;13:105–18.

34. WHO (World Health Organization). 2012. Depression http://www.who.int/topics/depression/en/. Accessed Feb 2015.

35. Castle DJ. Mental health histories and psychiatric medication usage among persons who sought cosmetic surgery (discussion). 223. Plast Reconstr Surg. 2004;114:1934.

36. Stevens L, McGrath MH. Psychological aspects of plastic surgery. In: Mathes SJ, editor. Plastic surgery, vol. 1. Philadelphia: Saunders; 2006. p. 67–91.

37. Del Aguila E, Pablos JL, Huanuco M, Encina VM, Rhenals AL. Personality traits, anxiety and self-esteem in patients seeking cosmetic surgery in Mexico City. Plast Reconstr Surgery Glob Open, 2019;1.

38. Renato de Paula P, Calixto Fortes de Arrudo F, Prado M, Gustavo Neves C. Prevalence of depressive symptoms in patients requesting cosmetic breast surgery in midwestern Brazil. Plast Reconstr Surg Glob Open. 2018;6(10)

39. Anxiety. https://en.wikipedia.org/wiki/Anxiety.

The Association of Breast Augmentation with Silicone Implants with Suicide

7

7.1   Introduction

Breast augmentation (augmentation mammoplasty) is the surgery performed to increase size, change the shape, and alter the texture of the breasts of a woman. It was the most common cosmetic procedure in 2018 with 313,735 operations performed which comprise a 48% increase since 2000 [1]. The increasing popularity of breast procedures can be explained by the importance that women attribute to the appearance of their breasts since antiquity. Breasts represent a woman's femininity, sensuality, and fertility and frequently play a significant role in fashion, advertising, and media underlining its value for society [2].

Dissatisfaction with the size and shape of someone's breasts is the prime motivation of women undergoing breast augmentation [3]. Additionally, women who wish to undergo the procedure declare that they want to feel more feminine, to be less shy with men, and to boost a sense of womanliness [4]. Another motivational factor frequently mentioned in the medical literature is improving someone's self-esteem, feeling better in general [5].

Augmentation has been traditionally performed with implants filled either with viscous silicone gel or sterile saline solution. Breast implants are placed in a subglandular, submuscular, or dual-plane pocket, with regard to their relationship to pectoralis major muscle. A more recent alternative technique is the fat graft transfer,

© Springer Nature Switzerland AG 2020

P. Milothridis, *Cosmetic Patient Selection and Psychosocial Background*,

https://doi.org/10.1007/978-3-030-44725-0_7

according to which augmentation is achieved with autologous adipocyte fat tissue, drawn from the woman's body. Its main advantage is that someone's own fat is used instead of any medical device.

Both techniques of elective breast augmentation result in improved psychological outcomes which have been constantly reported in medical literature. There is a significant and profoundly positive effect on women's satisfaction with their breasts, along with their quality of life and sexual well-being [6]. Women who have had cosmetic breast implants postoperatively report high overall satisfaction and experience good outcomes in psychosocial terms [7].

Despite the popularity of breast augmentation, the procedure has been and remains under intense scrutiny. Silicone implants have been among the most notorious medical devices ever used. They have been accused to cause various types of cancer and autoimmune diseases. More recently, many health policy leaders have posed concerns about the safety of breast implants that have heightened with the European Poly Implant Prothese implant crisis and the potential link of implants to anaplastic large cell lymphoma [8].

The conflict regarding safety of breast augmentation recently shifted toward its psychological impact. Despite the robust evidence about postoperative improvement in quality of life, women who have had cosmetic breast implants seem to have a two to three times increased risk of suicide [9]. The present challenge is to determine the predisposing factors of this risk and develop a clinical tool to identify the women who will benefit the less from the procedure.

7.2   Elective Breast Augmentation

Breast augmentation, sometimes referred to as a "breast aug" or "boob job" by patients, involves using breast implants or fat transfer to increase the size of breasts. Its history goes back to the late nineteenth century, when breast implants were first used to augment the size and modify breast shape. In 1895, surgeon Vincenz Czerny accomplished the earliest mammoplasty with implant when he used the patient's autologous adipose tissue, harvested from a benign lumbar lipoma, to repair the asymmetry of the breast from which he had removed a tumor. In 1889, surgeon Robert Gersuny experimented with paraffin injections with disastrous results.

The breakthrough of the procedure came with the development of silicone gel breast implants filled either with viscous silicone or saline solution. Its popularity increases steadily making it the most common cosmetic procedure in 2018.

The efficacy of breast implants has been documented via validated quality of life measurement tools such as the BREAST-Q. Elective breast augmentation offers significant improvements in women's satisfaction with breasts, psychosocial, and sexual well-being that persisted from the early postoperative period to at least 6 months afterward. Breast augmentation also has a very large magnitude of effect across all patient quality of life domains in both early and postoperative periods, except for physical functioning [10, 11].

The psychosocial benefits include greatly improved confidence in social setting, feelings of attractiveness, and self-assurance. Confidence with sexual activity and feelings of sexual attractiveness are significantly improved. Patients undergoing the procedure are also significantly more satisfied with their breast appearance, size, softness, and amount of cleavage.

However, these benefits can be compromised because of postoperative complications such as infection, pain, hematoma, silicone implant hemorrhage, capsular contracture, and loss of nipple sensation. These commonly result to revision surgeries which are performed, when the patient is unsatisfied with the outcome of the augmentation or when technical or medical complications occur. Revision rates are up to 20%, as reported by the US FDA [12].

7.3   Breast Implants

Augmentation mammoplasty was advanced with the introduction of silicone breast implants in the early 1960s. Breast implants are the prostheses used to change the size, shape, and contour of a person's breast. They are some of the most common medical devices used. In 2011, there were ten million women worldwide with breast implants [13]. They are categorized by their filler material, either silicone gel or saline solution. Alternative composition implants featured miscellaneous fillers such as soy oil and polypropylene string but are not recommended anymore due to safety concerns.

The first silicone implant was invented in 1961 by the American plastic surgeons Thomas Cronin and Frank Gerow. During the following years, technological developments have led to improvements of their safety and efficacy profile. However, in the early 1990s, the national health ministries of various countries reviewed published studies about causal links among silicone gel implants and systemic and autoimmune diseases. The US Food and Drug Administration, in response to these reports, decided a moratorium on the use of silicone gel implants in 1992. Moratorium was widespread by the media and resulted in dramatic decrease of women presenting for breast augmentation. This is now called the "implant crisis" of the 1990s.

During the following years, there had been no evidence to establish a causal connection between the implantation of implant and development of systemic disease, and popularity of the procedure has increased steadily in the postcrisis era.

Despite the number of studies demonstrating the safety of breast implants, patients remain reluctant especially about their possible association with malignancy. In fact, implants may interfere with the mammographic visualization of lesions, and there has been some evidence of a later presentation of disease among women with implants [14]. However, this should not be a problem in the hands of an experienced radiologist.

These concerns were examined thoroughly by large cohort studies. Breast augmentation patients show lower rates of deaths than the general population [15]. This is true even in the case of breast cancer, most likely reflecting that these patients have better access to medical care.

This is not relevant for anaplastic large cell lymphoma (ALCL), an extremely rare type of cancer. Breast implant-associated ALCL (BI-ALCL) is a distinctive T cell lymphoma that arises around breast implants. The risk of developing BI-ALCL is significantly higher than developing ALCL in the general population. BI-ALCL appears to develop just over 10 years from the time of implant placement, and the reported lifetime prevalence is 1 in 30,000 women with textured breast implants [16].

Regarding other types of malignancy, respiratory cancers were more frequently observed among breast implant patients. Researchers attributed their finding to higher rates of smoking [17]. Similarly, higher rates of death because of motor vehicle accidents may be attributed to alcohol or drug exposures. The abovementioned data underscore the contribution of patients' personality characteristics to their long-term outcome.

The main reason for the placement of moratorium in 1992 was to clarify any association between silicone implants and the development of autoimmune diseases such as scleroderma, systematic erythematic lupus, mixed disorders of the connective tissue, rheumatoid arthritis, and Sjogren's syndrome. Lack of robust evidence to confirm any association led to removal of any restriction. However, a recent report suggests that silicone implantation for more than 10 years in women with hyperimmune state or atopy may cause autoimmune syndrome induced by adjuvants (ASIA) [18]. Clinical manifestations of ASIA are fatigue, night sweats, morning stiffness, and joint and muscle pain.

Similarly, fibromyalgia syndrome is a more common chronic condition which has been associated with silicone implants [19]. It is characterized by generalized musculoskeletal pain and low levels of 5-hydroxyindoleacetic acid (5-HIAA) in cerebrospinal fluid. This biomarker has been identified as a possible suicide risk predictor [20]. A large-scale study examining outcomes of nearly 100 thousand women with breast implants concluded that silicone implants are linked to the development of connective tissue diseases (CTDs) and patient-reported rheumatoid symptoms [21]. The great number of limitations of the latter and other similar studies makes any association of silicone implants with autoimmune diseases uncertain.

7.4   Psychosocial Profile of Breast Augmentation Patients

The demographic, psychosocial, and behavioral characteristics of women undergoing breast augmentation must be clarified when examining long-term outcomes. The main factor that motivates women to seek breast augmentation is the dissatisfaction from the appearance of their breast that subsequently leads to avoidance of being seen undressed and constantly wearing camouflaging outfits [22]. These women have poor romantic and interpersonal relationships because of their body image concerns [23].

Breasts have been an eternal symbol of femininity and fertility since the Paleolithic era as depicted through the sculptural work of that time. Nowadays, the leading motivation of modern women to seek augmentation mammoplasty is improvement of their well-being and femininity. Solvi et al. [24] studied the Serbian augmentation mammoplasty candidates and found that their basic drive was to feel more feminine.

However, not every woman desires the procedure. Several studies have defined the demographic characteristics of breast augmentation patients. They are predominantly Caucasian and range in age from 20 to 49 [25]. Regarding marital status, there is a greater tendency for breast augmentation candidates to be single and have middle to upper socioeconomic status. Cook et al. [26] reported that 28.8% of breast augmentation patients were divorced or separated relative to 18.1% in the comparison group. However, other studies remain inconclusive regarding their marital status. Evidence by two Scandinavian studies [27, 28] suggests that rates of current smoking among breast augmentation patients are close to two times the rate among the general population. Additionally, these women consume large amounts of alcohol at higher rates [26]. Other characteristics cited in the literature include a wide variety of qualities, some favorable and others not so. Increased rates of gynecologic problems and sexual dysfunction have been described in patients presenting for breast augmentation [4, 26].

A conflicting study demonstrated that breast augmentation patients reported more positive sexual functioning compared with a matched control group [29]. Generally, breast augmentation patients are found to invest more time and effort into health and fitness concerns. Breast augmentation women are more likely to have had an induced abortion and show greater number of full pregnancies, more sexual partners, and earlier age at the time of first childbirth [26]. All these features represent indirect indexes of impulsivity. Other personality disorders may also be common among women with breast implants.

Even though psychopathology is uncommon among augmentation mammoplasty patients, dissatisfaction with their breasts may occasionally be correlated with depressive symptoms. They have been shown to demonstrate varying degrees of low self-esteem, anxiety, and depression. Interestingly, a recent study found a higher prevalence of psychiatric admissions before cosmetic surgery among women undergoing breast implant surgeries than among women undergoing breast reduction or other cosmetic surgery procedures [30]. Another study demonstrated that the incidence of depressive symptoms among cosmetic patients is higher among women with breast implants. The prevalence of depressive symptoms (DS) was found in 18.9% of cosmetic breast surgery patients [31], and women who presented in public institutions have a 2.3 times greater risk of having DS than those presented in private institutions. This finding should be taken into consideration by doctors working in public hospitals, as it suggests that their patients' psychosocial characteristics may differ from those in private sector.

Table 7.1 Risk factors for suicide in general population

Current ideation, intent, plan, access to means
Previous suicide attempt
Alcohol/substance abuse
Current or previous history of psychiatric diagnosis
Impulsivity and poor self-control
Hopelessness—Presence, duration, personal
Recent discharge from an inpatient psychiatric unit
Family history of suicide
History of abuse (physical, sexual, or emotional)
Comorbid health problems (new diagnosis or worsening symptoms)
Age, gender, race (elderly or young adult, unmarried, white, male, who lives alone)
Same-sex sexual orientation

7.5   The Social Burden of Suicide

Suicide is a major, preventable public health problem. Approximately 0.5% of people die of suicide [32], and Europe had the highest rates by region in 2015 [33]. Suicide has been correlated with many factors, including family history of suicide, conduct disorders, depressive disorders, anxiety states, alcoholism, and drug abuse. Triggering factors may include acute stress, trouble with the law, pregnancy or fear of pregnancy, social isolation, anxiety, and environmental change [34]. The risk factors for suicide in general population according to the National Institute of Mental Health in the United States are stated in Table 7.1.

Women of age range 35–44 years who are unmarried, divorced, or single without social support and with occupational instability are of high risk for suicide [35]. Infertility and miscarriage have also been linked to increase risk especially when induced [36].

7.6   Association Between Breast Augmentation with Implants and Suicide

Lifetime risk of suicide among women with breast implants seems to be two to three times higher than among those without. In medical literature, there are six epidemiological cohort studies addressing the issue of cosmetic breast augmentation and suicide [15, 17, 30, 37–39]. This finding has caused a conflict regarding the safety of cosmetic breast augmentation and has led to many empirical explanations [40]. However, the studies which demonstrated an increased risk for suicide in augmentation patients fail to identify a cause-and-effect relationship [9].

The increased risk is more likely to be attributed to breast augmentation patients' psychosocial features. Characteristics that would increase their risk for suicide compared with the general population include alcohol and drug abuse, smoking, and single marital status. Joiner [41] calculated that the risk of the prototypical breast augmentation women to commit suicide would be approximately four times higher than that of general population. He estimated the expected suicide rate based on their age, race, divorced status, smoking habits, alcohol abuse, impulsivity, and depressive symptoms.

The strongest and most consistently reported risk factor for suicide appears to be previous hospitalization for psychiatric reasons [39]. Therefore, plastic surgeons have to obtain a psychiatric history in terms of the preoperative consultation. Direct questions about outpatient treatment or past psychiatric consultations should be made. Generally, 20% of cosmetic patients report ongoing psychiatric treatment, most commonly the use of antidepressants [42]. When plastic surgeons believe that psychiatric symptoms are not well controlled, referral to a psychiatrist is necessary. This is consistent with recommendations for the management of the high-risk patient for suicide [43].

Patient age was also found to be significantly associated with satisfaction outcomes following breast augmentation, with diminished satisfaction with advanced age. Older patients seem less satisfied with their aesthetic result and less likely to have their expectations met [10]. This is consistent with the finding that the highest risk for suicide was observed among women who received their implants at 40 years of age or older [15].

In terms of the elevated risk of suicide among breast augmentation patients during their lifetime, plastic surgeons have to schedule long-term post-op visits. It has been shown that the result of suicide among women with breast implants was not elevated in the first 10 years of follow-up but was increased in all subsequent time periods [15]. Therefore, it is important to never lose contact with breast implant patients. Complications and increased risk for suicide are more likely to occur in a longer than 10-year time period.

7.7 Clinical Tool

Suicide prediction is a complex task. A combination of demographic variables, psychiatric history, and social, biological, and other factors must be evaluated individually and in the context of the patient's whole environment [44]. The risk factors should not be considered independently, because this can result in prediction errors. Nevertheless, plastic surgeons have to take into considerations the risk factors that may predispose their breast implant patients to suicide.

Based on medical literature, increased risk for suicide following breast augmentation is linked with previous hospitalization for psychiatric reasons and with age older than 40 years. A combination of these two characteristics during preoperative consultation is an alarming sign that indicates referral to a mental health professional.

Other risk factors for suicide in general population have to be clarified. Alcohol and substance abuse, depressive symptoms, current use of psychiatric medication,

Fig. 7.1 High-risk breast
augmentation patient

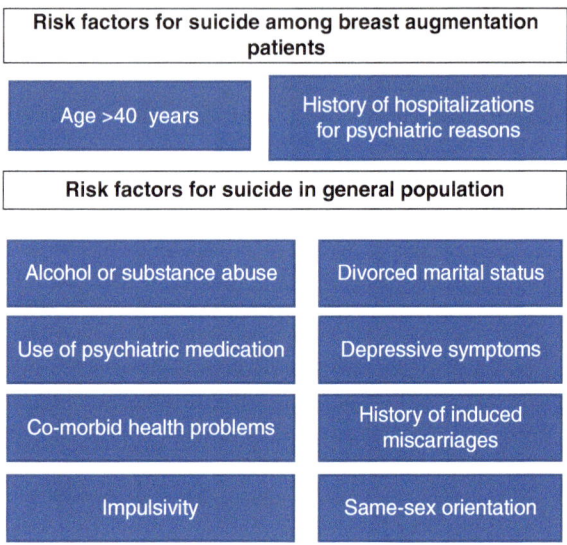

same-sex orientation, divorced marital status, comorbid serious health problems, and impulsivity have to be taken into consideration during preoperative consultation.

These characteristics may prove helpful for plastic surgeons, as better understanding of cosmetic breast patients leads to improved health-care service (Fig. 7.1). Women with the abovementioned characteristics should not be immediately excluded from breast augmentation. Every case should be examined individually. Close collaboration between plastic surgeons and the mental health professionals is mandatory [45].

7.8   Conclusion

Breast augmentation is beneficial for women in terms of improvement of various aspects of quality of life. However, there is a two to three times increased suicide risk among these patients. This can be attributed to their psychosocial characteristics. A clinical tool is developed to assist plastic surgeons in the selection of breast augmentation patients during preoperative consultation.

References

1. ASPS statistics report. https://www.plasticsurgery.org/documents/News/Statistics/2018/plastic-surgery-statistics-report-2018.pdf.
2. Yalom MA. History of the breast. New York: Knopf; 1997.
3. Sarwer DB. The psychological aspects of cosmetic breast augmentation. Plast Reconstr Surg. 2007;120:110e7.
4. Birtchnell S, Whitfield P, Lacey JH. Motivational factors in women requesting augmentation and reduction mammoplasty. J Psychosom Res. 1990;34:509e14.

5. Ferraro GA, Rossano F, D'Andrea F. Self-perception and self-esteem of patients seeking cosmetic surgery. Aesthet Plast Surg. 2005;29:184e9.
6. McCarthy CM, Cano SJ, Klassen AF, Scott A, van Laeken N, Lennox PA, Cordeiro PG, Pusic AL. The magnitude of effect of cosmetic breast augmentation on patient satisfaction and health-related quality of life. Plast Reconstr Surg. 2012;130:218–23.
7. Cash TF, Duel LA, Perkins LL. Women's psychosocial outcomes of breast augmentation with silicone gel-filled implants: a 2-year prospective study. Plast Reconstr Surg. 2002;109(6):2122–3.
8. U.S. Food and Drug Administration. FDA review indicates possible association between breast implants and a rare cancer. 2011. http://www.fda.gov/NewsEvents/Newsroom/PressAnnouncements/ucm241090.htm. Accessed 21 July 2010.
9. Rohrich RJ, Adams WP Jr, Potter JK. A review of psychological outcomes and suicide in aesthetic breast augmentation. Plast Reconstr Surg. 2007;119(1):401–8.
10. Alderman AK, Bauer J, Fardo D, Abrahamse P, Pusic A. Understanding the effect of breast augmentation on quality of life: prospective analysis using the BREAST-Q. Plast Reconstr Surg. 2014;133(4):787–95.
11. Coriddi M, Angelos T, Nadeau M, Bennett M, Taylor A. Analysis of satisfaction and Well-being in the short follow-up from breast augmentation using the BREAST-Q, a validated survey instrument. Aesthet Surg J. 2013;33:245–51.
12. Tebbetts JB. Out points criteria for breast implant removal without replacement and criteria to minimize reoperations following breast augmentation. Plast Reconstr Surg. 2006;114(5):1258–62.
13. FDA Implants and Prostheses. http://www.fda.gov/MedicalDevices/ProductsandMedicalProcedures/ImplantsandProsthetics/BreastImplants/ucm239996.htm. Published January 2011. Accessed Mar 2019.
14. Silverstein MJ, Handel N, Gamagami P, Gierson ED, Furmanski M, Collins AR, Epstein M, Cohlan BF. Breast cancer diagnosis and prognosis in women following augmentation with silicone gel-filled prostheses. Eur J Cancer. 1992;28:635–40.
15. Brinton LA, Lubin JH, Murray MC, et al. Mortality rates among augmentation mammoplasty patients: an update. Epidemiology. 2006;164:334–41.
16. Doren EL, Miranda RN, Selber JC, Garvey PB, Liu J, Medeiros LJ, Clemens MW. U.S. epidemiology of breast implant-associated anaplastic large cell lymphoma. Plast Reconstr Surg. 2017;139(5):1042–50.
17. Koot VC, Peeters PH, Granath F, Grobbee DE, Nyren O. Total and cause specific mortality among Swedish women with cosmetic breast implants: prospective study. BMJ. 2003;326:527–8.
18. Maijers MC, de Blok CJ, Niessen FB, van der Veidt AA, Ritt MJ, Winters HA, Kramer MH, Nanayakkara PW. Women with silicone breast implants and unexplained systemic symptoms: a descriptive cohort study. Neth J Med. 2013;71:534–40.
19. Richards S, Cleare AJ. Fibromyalgia: biological correlates. Curr Opin Psychiatry. 2000;13:623–8.
20. Arango V, Huang YY, Underwood MD, Mann JJ. Genetics of the serotonergic system in suicidal behavior. J Psychiatr Res. 2003;37:375–86.
21. Coroneos CJ, Selber JC, Offodile AC 2nd, Butler CE, Clemens MW. US FDA breast implant postapproval studies: long-term outcomes in 99,993 patients. Ann Surg. 2019;269(1):30–6.
22. Sarwer DB, Pertschuk MJ, Wadden TA, Whitaker LA. Psychological investigations in cosmetic surgery: a look-back and a look ahead. Plast Reconstr Surg. 1998;101(4):1136–42.
23. Sarwer DB, Whitaker LA, Pertschuk MJ, Wadden TA. Body image concerns of reconstructive surgery patients: an underrecognized problem. Ann Plast Surg. 1998;40(4):403–7.
24. Solvi AS, Foss K, von Soest T, Roald HE, Skolleborg KC, Holte A. Motivational factors and psychological processes in cosmetic breast augmentation surgery. J Plast Reconstr Aesthet Surg. 2018;63(4):673–80.
25. Brinton LA, Brown LS, Colton T, Burich MC, Lubin J. Characteristics of a population of women with breast implants compared with women seeking other types of plastic surgery. Plast Reconstr Surg. 2000;105:919–27.
26. Cook LS, Daling JR, Voigt LF, DeHart MP, Malone KE, Stanford JL, Weiss NS, Brinton LA, Gammon MD, Brogan D. Characteristics of women with and without breast augmentation. JAMA. 1997;277:1612–7.

27. Fryzek JP, Weiderpass E, Signorello LB, Hakelius L, Lipworth L, Blot WJ, McLaughlin JK, Nyren O. Characteristics of women with cosmetic breast augmentation surgery compared with breast reduction surgery patients and women in the general population of Sweden. Ann Plast Surg. 2000;45:349–56.
28. Kjoller K, Holmich LR, Fryzek JP, Jacobsen PH, Friis S, McLaughlin JK, Lipworth L, Henriksen TF, Jorgensen S, Bittman S, Olsen JH. Characteristics of women with cosmetic breast implants compared with women with other types of cosmetic surgery and population-based controls in Denmark. Ann Plast Surg. 2003;50:6–12.
29. Didie ER, Sarwer DB. Factors that influence the decision to undergo cosmetic breast augmentation surgery. J Women's Health. 2003;12:241.
30. Jacobsen PH, Holmich LR, McLaughlin JK, Johansen C, Olsen JH, Kholler K, Friis S. Mortality and suicide among Danish women with cosmetic breast implants. Arch Intern Med. 2004;164:2450–5.
31. Renato de Paula P, Calixto Fortes de Arrudo F, Prado M, Gustavo Neves C. Prevalence of depressive symptoms in patients requesting cosmetic breast surgery in midwestern Brazil. Plast Reconstr Surg Glob Open. 2018;6(10)
32. Chang B, Gitlin D, Patel R. The depressed and suicidal patient in the emergency department: evidenced-based management and treatment strategies. Emerg Med Pract. 13(9):1–23.
33. World Health Organization. Suicide rates per. https://www.who.int/gho/mental_health/suicide_rates_crude/en/.
34. Irwin CE, Shafer MA. Adolescent health problems. In: Harrison's principles of internal medicine. 13th ed. New York: McGraw-Hill; 1994.
35. Samandari G, Martin SL, Kupper LL, Schiro S, Norwood T, Avery M. Are pregnant and post-partum women: at increased risk for violent death? Suicide and homicide findings from North Carolina. Matern Child Health J. 2011;15:660–9.
36. Gissler M, Hemminki E, Lonnqvist J. Suicides after pregnancy in Finland, 1987-94: register linkage study. BMJ. 1996;313:1431–4.
37. Pukkala E, Kulmala I, Hovi SL, Hemminski E, Keskimaki I, Pakkanen M, Lipworth L, Boice JD Jr, McLaughlin JK. Causes of death among Finnish women with cosmetic breast implants, 1971-2001. Ann Plast Surg. 2003;51:339–42.
38. Villeneuve PJ, Holowaty EJ, Brisson J, Xie L, Ugnat AM, Latulippe L, Mao Y. Mortality among Canadian women with cosmetic breast implants. Am J Epidemiol. 2006;164:334–41.
39. Lipworth L, Nyren O, Ye W, Fryzek JP, Tarone RE, McLaughlin JK. Excess mortality from suicide and other external causes of death among women with cosmetic breast implants. Ann Plast Surg. 2007;59(2):119–23.
40. Morgan E. Suicide after breast augmentation. Epidemiology. 2008;19:520–1.
41. Joiner T. Does breast augmentation confer risk of or protection from suicide? Aesthet Surg J. 2003;23(5):370–5.
42. Sarwer DB, Zanville HA, LaRossa D, Bartlett SP, Chang B, Low DW, Whitaker LA. Mental health histories and psychiatric medication usage among persons who sought cosmetic surgery. Plast Reconstr Surg. 2004;114:1927–33.
43. Goldsmith SK, Pellmar TC, Kleinman AM, Bunney WE. Reducing suicide: a National Imperative. Washington, DC: National Academy Press; 2002.
44. Manoloudakis N, Labiris G, Karakitsou N, Kim JB, Sheena Y, Niakas D. Characteristics of women who have had cosmetic breast implants that could be associated with increased suicide risk: a systematic review, proposing a suicide prevention model. Arch Plast Surg. 2015;42(2):131–42.
45. Sarwer DB. Psychological assessment of cosmetic surgery patients. In: Sarwer DB, Pruzinsky T, Cash TF, Goldwyn RM, Persing JA, Whitaker LA, editors. Psychological aspects of reconstructive and cosmetic plastic surgery: empirical, clinical, and ethical issues. Philadelphia: Lippincott Williams & Wilkins; 2006. p. 267–83.

Psychosocial Assessment of the Rhinoplasty Candidate: The DUMPO Profile

Definitions

Aesthetic means concerned with beauty or the appreciation of beauty.

Body dysmorphic disorder is a psychiatric disorder consisting of distressing or impairing preoccupation with a nonexistent or slight defect in someone's appearance.

Rhinoplasty is a surgical procedure that alters the shape or appearance of the nose while preserving or enhancing the nasal airway. The primary reason for surgery can be aesthetic, functional, or both and may include adjunctive procedures on the septum, turbinates, or paranasal sinuses.

8.1 Introduction

Rhinoplasty is the surgical procedure that alters the appearance of the nose while preserving or enhancing the nasal airway. According to the American Society of Plastic Surgeons, nose reshaping was the third most popular cosmetic surgical procedure in 2017, with 218,924 rhinoplasty procedures performed [1].

Its popularity can be attributed to the central position of the nose in the face. Correction of nasal deformities contributes to the overall beauty and attractiveness. Additionally, it has been found that aesthetic rhinoplasty improves the public perception of a patient's personality [2]. People evaluated postoperative photos of rhinoplasty patients as more likeable, trustworthy, confident, approachable, and intelligent. Interestingly, an alteration in appearance following a rhinoplasty alters social perception about the patient.

Surgical rhinoplasty is one of the most technically and artistically challenging procedures in the purview of cosmetic surgery. Changes to nasal anatomy require advanced skills with manipulation of the bone, cartilage, and skin. It is a matter of millimeters to make an error which will have a negative impact on both appearance

© Springer Nature Switzerland AG 2020
P. Milothridis, *Cosmetic Patient Selection and Psychosocial Background*,
https://doi.org/10.1007/978-3-030-44725-0_8

and function. Scar formation following nose reshaping is unpredictable and may alter the outcome several months postoperatively. So, it is commonly stated that rhinoplasty is an easy operation to perform but a difficult one to achieve an outstanding result.

Except for the technical difficulties, physicians have the challenging task of patient selection because some candidates are unsuitable for treatment. Some argue that cosmetic rhinoplasty patients are psychologically unstable compared to other patients and therefore a "risky" group to operate [3]. Nose is the predominant facial feature; thus, nasal aesthetic deformities may be associated with significant body image dissatisfaction. For the same reason, rhinoplasty is exposed to significant critical analysis because the results are so obvious.

Despite these drawbacks, aesthetic nasal surgery can be of tremendous benefit toward improving self-esteem and quality of life. To select the optimal rhinoplasty candidates, physicians should consider functional, aesthetic, and psychological components. Patients should be assessed for the ability to set achievable goals. This is very important, as candidates with unrealistic expectations may be dissatisfied from the procedure. This will lead to cosmetic physician's potential physical, emotional, and financial injury inflicted by problematic patients. Despite the popularity and importance of rhinoplasty, there are currently no evidence-based clinical tools to optimize patient selection.

8.2   Nonsurgical Rhinoplasty

Traditionally, rhinoplasty has been performed by ear-nose-throat (ENT) surgeons and maxillofacial and plastic surgeons to permanently restore aesthetic deformities and reconstruct the nasal airway. Although the surgical technique remains the gold standard of treatment, many candidates are concerned about the long recovery period with swelling and bruises, as well as the risk that general anesthesia carries.

Minimally invasive rhinoplasty using injectable fillers offers low morbidity, unimpaired skin quality and texture, cost-effectiveness, and quick recovery, making this option an emerging tool in the aesthetic medicine that deserves special focus. Injectable fillers are a viable alternative to surgery with minimal downtime and high satisfaction rates [4].

Its popularity is constantly increasing, and dermatologists and cosmetic doctors perform nonsurgical rhinoplasties in their medical offices. Thus, optimal selection of the rhinoplasty patients is a clinical task of both surgical and nonsurgical medical specialties.

8.3   The High-Risk Rhinoplasty Patient

Some patients will prove to be unhappy regardless of an apparently successful rhinoplasty, and physicians should exclude them from receiving treatment. Some physicians' decision is based on their instinct and an unclear feeling of disliking the patient. However, this subjective approach may be biased, and clinical tools should be applied during the first consultation.

Gorney sets out the "red flag characteristics" of a rhinoplasty patient [5]. The acronym SIMON (*s*ingle, *i*mmature, *m*ale, *o*verly expectant, *n*arcissist) was coined for the male high-risk patient. Rhinoplasty patients who are characterized by these five features have been thought to be potentially problematic with lower postoperative satisfaction rates. The SIMON profile has been a well-known clinical tool for physicians to assess the rhinoplasty candidates and select the ones who will benefit the most from the procedure. However, reviewing medical literature about negative predictors of satisfaction following postoperative satisfaction suggests that it may be not entirely evidenced-based.

8.4   SIMON: S (Single)

Many rhinoplasty candidates are young and single. Even though that single marital status is a common demographic characteristic of the rhinoplasty candidate, there is no published data to support that being single may influence the satisfaction rate following the procedure. Rhinoplasty is popular among young individuals, and physicians should not be preoccupied that marital status is a predictor of its outcome.

8.5   SIMON: I (Immature)

Maturity has a dual meaning being defined either as a person's mental competence or the state of being fully grown. In medical literature, there is no data to support that immaturity from the perspective of emotional childishness is a negative predictor of rhinoplasty outcome. However, age below 30 years is a characteristic that is associated with poor satisfaction rates. Results of unhappy rhinoplasty patients showed a great likelihood of dissatisfaction in younger male patients (average age: 29.4 years) [6]. To be more accurate, age below 30 rather than the level of maturity is a factor that can predict poor outcome following rhinoplasty.

8.6   SIMON: M (Male)

Male sex has been described as a negative predictor for satisfaction following rhinoplasty. Male patients tend to have relatively nonspecific complaints and are typically more demanding. In general, they have a poorer understanding of the deformity than women [7]. Furthermore, they tend to have a more difficult time describing the changes they think are needed and are much less attentive during consultations [8]. Indeed, the percentage of satisfaction following rhinoplasty has been found to be three times greater in **women** than in **men** ($p < 0.01$) [6]. This can be explained by the unique psychological characteristics of the average male rhinoplasty candidate. He seems to feel an above average amount of anxiety and depression than other men and has been described as having "female sensitivities for quality of appearance" [9]. Male sex is a risk factor that has to be considered during the first consultation.

8.7   SIMON: O (Overly Expectant)

Having unrealistic expectations is one of the most often described factors regarding disappointing results after cosmetic facial surgery. Overly expectant patients often request a total makeover of their nose with instantly recognizable positive results. In fact, there is swelling especially on the tip following open rhinoplasty, and the final cosmetic result is obvious after several months. This is something that patients should be well informed about; otherwise, their great expectations may cause discomfort during the postoperative period.

Even the most skilled rhinoplasty surgeons occasionally have suboptimal results. This is explained by the unique nasal anatomy which can be easily distorted by unpredictable scar formation and must be explained to and understood by the patients during the first consultation. Rhinoplasty candidates with high expectations who do not seem to understand the unpredictable nature of the procedure are thought to be problematic patients with low satisfaction rates [10].

Another aspect of the overly expectant patients is that they cannot describe their problem in detail. When the physician asks what exactly they are worried about, they do not seem to have a clear understanding of their deformities. They visit the office with photographs of celebrities to explain what adjustment they want and request a similar postoperative result. Generally, they seek perfection but are not able to express what kind of improvements they need.

Management of the overly expectant patient is manifested in a major guideline of aesthetic rhinoplasty clinical practice:

"Clinicians should ask all patients seeking rhinoplasty about their motivations for surgery and their expectations for outcomes, should provide feedback on whether those expectations are a realistic goal for surgery, and should document this discussion in the medical record" [11]. This guideline highlights the importance of educating patients during the consultation and selecting the ones who have realistic demands.

8.8   Motivation and Secondary Gain

Cosmetic patients should have an inner motivation to change their appearance and improve their psychosocial well-being and quality of life. However, there are occasionally external factors like friends, partners, or other family members who urge cosmetic candidates to change their appearance. Externally directed motivation is notorious to produce poor results. Cosmetic patients should be self-motivated and not driven by the desire to please someone else.

Another example of wrong motivational pattern is when the expectations of the surgical outcome do not have to do with improving their appearance but are closely related to success in, for instance, the job and relationships. This phenomenon is often referred to as "secondary gain" [12]. Evidence suggests that patients are more likely to view their surgery as a success if their motivation for surgery is self-improvement rather than expectations relating to external factors.

Life crises include divorce, loss of job, beloved persons, function by illness, or accident. Patients in crises may expect unrealistically that a positive change to their physical appearance will bring about positive changes in many aspects of their personal or professional lives.

These patients should be rejected during the selection process at least until they are more stable. This may entail waiting 6 to 12 months after the inciting event or until the stressful situation or grief resolves. Initially, a referral to a psychologist or psychiatrist is indicated as assistance to adapt to the new situation or achieve self-awareness. Later, these patients may become good candidates for cosmetic surgery.

Clinical Pearls: Patients' Motivation
- *Assess patients' expectations and understanding of the unpredictability of the results.*
- *What changes exactly would they like you to perform?*
- *Is there anyone in their environment who suggested them to undergo the procedure?*
- *Do they believe that rhinoplasty could improve your marriage, career, or relationships?*

8.9   SIMON: N (Narcissistic)

A narcissistic personality disorder is a disorder with a long-term pattern of abnormal behavior characterized by exaggerated feelings of self-importance, excessive need for admiration, and a lack of empathy. Those affected often spend much time thinking about achieving power or success or on their appearance [13]. It has been found to be the most common personality trait of people who are interested in rhinoplasty [14]. However, it has not described as a negative predictor of satisfaction following rhinoplasty since 1975 [15]. On the contrary, patients with obsessive-compulsive and antisocial personality disorders have lower satisfaction rate among rhinoplasty patients [16].

8.10   Body Dysmorphic Disorder (BDD)

Interview-based studies performed in the 1950s to 1960s reported that the majority of cosmetic surgery patients had some form of significant psychological pathology, but this opinion seems to be outdated. Merely having or having had a mental illness should not of itself preclude cosmetic procedures. An exception of this is considered to be body dysmorphic disorder (BDD).

BDD is a psychiatric disorder that appears in the Diagnostic and Statistical Manual of Mental Disorders under the section of obsessive-compulsive and related disorders [17]. It is an independent risk factor for lower satisfaction following rhinoplasty. BDD patients are specifically obsessed with nonexistent or minimal flaws or defects in their appearance, which are typically not observable or appear slight to others. Any part of the body may be the focus of concern in body dysmorphic disorder, but the most common areas involved are the skin, hair, and nose [18].

Patients with BDD typically express concern about the appearance of their nose and seek cosmetic surgery or minimally invasive procedures to improve it. The prevalence of moderate to severe BBD symptoms among rhinoplasty candidates has been found to be 33% [19]. Perception of the problem by patients is inaccurate because dissatisfaction with the nose is a product of the mental disorder, but the defect is perceived on their face. Consequently, they usually seek physical instead of psychiatric interventions.

These concerns can be remarkably stressful and are associated with symptoms that cause marked distress and life disruption. Every cosmetic surgeon should be aware that BDD symptoms may worsen following rhinoplasty, as patients become even more preoccupied with their perceived nasal deformity. They may seek more operative procedures or pursue other forms of rectification for their perceptions of failed surgery, e.g., injectable fillers. Therefore, BDD has been traditionally thought to be a contraindication for elective rhinoplasty.

However, some authors disagree that BDD is an absolute contraindication for aesthetic nasal surgery reasoning that the procedure could be beneficial for individuals with mild symptoms [20]. It seems that the severity of BDD plays a significant role in postoperative satisfaction rather than the presence of the syndrome itself. Indeed, it has been found that patients' benefit from rhinoplasty surgery is disproportionate to their preoperative obsession with their appearance.

Dissatisfaction with the size or shape of the nose may also be aggravated by sociocultural factors related to ethnicity, as the culturally dominant aesthetic standard places increased value on the Caucasian nose compared to variation associated with different ethnic groups [21]. So, any patient requesting an ethnic rhinoplasty in order to have a more "Caucasian-appearing" nose or presenting with a need to belong to a certain cultural group may suffer from BDD symptoms [22].

In terms of patient selection, it is the degree of preoperative symptoms of body dysmorphic disorder that determines postoperative satisfaction and quality of life in aesthetic rhinoplasty, and surgery may be indicated in the treatment of patients with mild to moderate BDD. The degree of body dissatisfaction in patients with BDD is associated with their degree of body image distortion, which affects their level of distress. The patient's level of distress may be the most important aspect in the diagnosis of BDD to be evaluated during the selection of cosmetic candidates [23], whereas patients with dysmorphophobia (severe BDD) should not receive a cosmetic intervention.

The finding that rhinoplasty may be not contraindicated to patients with mild to moderate BDD is important because it shows that a substantial number of patients who have been denied treatment based on their BDD may benefit from a cosmetic procedure to relieve their emotional distress.

8.11   Screening the BDD Rhinoplasty Candidate

Identifying the cosmetic patient with BDD is a challenging clinical task, as it is often present in a hidden state [24]. Assessment of BDD can be performed with the use of questionnaires, e.g., the Body Dysmorphic Symptom Scale [25]. Cutoff scores classify individuals who have mild, moderate, severe, or no BDD symptoms. Completion of a questionnaire during preoperative consultation of a cosmetic candidate is not always practical, as it may be stressful for the patient and time-consuming. However, the physician should be aware of signs, symptoms, and repetitive behaviors that could constitute a BDD diagnosis.

Clinical Pearls: Repetitive Behaviors
- *Checking repeatedly his/her nose at the mirror.*
- *Touching and palpating his/her nose, trying to elevate the tip or press down the dorsum.*
- *Asking questions about the present nasal appearance over and over again.*
- *Recalling emotionally past events or conversations about his/her nose.*
- *Comparing his/her nose to others (e.g., the physician's one).*
- *Contouring of the nose with excessive makeup.*
- *Seeking perfection. Their construction of thoughts and behavior are also based on perfectionism.*
- *Is there any functional impairment, for example, social avoidance, because of nasal appearance?*

If a rhinoplasty candidate presents with the abovementioned characteristics, cosmetic doctors should request for a psychiatric evaluation prior to the procedure.

8.12   Minimal Deformities

Seeking surgical intervention to restore a minimal nasal deformity is also a high-risk factor for postoperative satisfaction, as it may indicate a psychological imbalance. Female rhinoplasty candidates with greater nasal deformity have been found to have better mental health compared to the ones with minimal ones [26]. In such cases, seeking cosmetic intervention functions as a way to improve the psychological status or alleviate symptoms of anxiety or depression. However, a lesser degree of deformity with a simultaneously higher concern is an alarming combination in the selection of rhinoplasty patients.

Clinical Pearls
- *Assess the objective degree of nasal deformity and compare it to the patient's concern about it.*

8.13   History of Previous Operations

Secondary rhinoplasty has long been considered a challenging procedure, and patients seeking this operation tend to be difficult to please [27]. Scar formation and deformities caused by bad technique during primary rhinoplasty like polly-beak, inverted-V, or pinch deformity raise the level of difficulty of the secondary procedure and should be considered preoperatively.

Except for the technical difficulties, the rhinoplasty specialist should probably be most concerned about the psychological aspects of the secondary rhinoplasty patient. Individuals who have had numerous procedures performed by many practitioners, and particularly those who report the outcome of such procedures to have been unsatisfactory, are notorious to be problematic. Patients who are disappointed with apparently successful results are called "surgiholics" [10]. Any history of legal proceedings or threats or overt violence toward previous cosmetic surgeons should be obviously considered very worrisome. These patients typically idealize the surgeon expecting him or her to accomplish what others had failed to do.

"Surgiholics" often try to compensate for a poor body image or even more serious psychological problems [28]. They tend to be fully informed about the latest surgical trends, and they have a fairly educated concept of exactly what they expect the surgeon to improve. These psychosocial characteristics in addition to the anatomical difficulties of the operated nose comprise a negative predictor of satisfaction following rhinoplasty.

Clinical Pearls: "Surgiholics"
- *Already operated patients with objectively good results who are still dissatisfied.*
- *Patients informed about the latest advances in cosmetic medicine.*
- *Patients who suggest themselves technical approaches to restore their problem.*
- *Idealization of the physician with phrases like "you are the best," "I am so lucky I found you," and "I wish I had met you earlier".*
- *History of legal proceedings to their previous physicians.*

Given the abovementioned evidenced-based characteristics of the high-risk rhinoplasty patient, it is evident that SIMON profile is partially evidenced-based. During the preoperative consultation, a rhinoplasty physician should be concerned about:

- **D**ysmorphophobia signs in.
- **U**nder 30 years old.
- **M**ale patients who had.
- **P**revious rhinoplasty with objectively good results and are.
- **O**verly expectant about outcome.

The DUMPO profile comprises an acronym with the five main characteristics of the high-risk rhinoplasty patients. A second preoperative consultation may be needed to review the patient's desire, develop a realistic operative plan, and confirm the patient's understanding of the anticipated procedure. After the second consultation, the rhinoplasty physician may decide to refer these patients to a psychiatrist, as they will probably not have significant satisfaction following the procedure. So, the DUMPO clinical tool may prove useful, as these patients should probably be DUMP-ed out during the selection process.

8.14   Conclusion

Rhinoplasty patient selection during the preoperative consultation is a challenging clinical task. The DUMPO profile may prove a useful tool to exclude high-risk candidates from treatment.

References

1. American Society of Plastic Surgeons. 2017 plastic surgery statistics report. https://www.plasticsurgery.org/news/press-releases/new-statistics-reveal-the-shape-of-plastic-surgery. Assessed 03 Mar 2019.
2. Lu SM, Hsu DT, Perry AD, Leipziger LS, Kasabian AK, Bartlett SP, Thome CH, Broer PN, Tanna N. The public face of Rhinoplasty. Impact on perceived attractiveness and personality. Plast Reconstr Surg. 2018;142(4):881–7.
3. Naraghi M, Atari M. Comparison of patterns of psychopathology in aesthetic rhinoplasty patients versus functional rhinoplasty patients. Otoralyngol Head Neck Surg. 2015;152(2):244–9.
4. Bertossi D, Lanaro L, Dorelan S, Johanssen K, Nocini P. Nonsurgical rhinoplasty: nasal grid analysis and nasal injecting protocol. Plast Reconstr Surg. 2019;143(2):428–39.
5. Gorney M. Criteria for patient selection: An ounce of prevention. Presented at the Residents and Fellows Forum, Aesthetic Plastic Surgery Annual Meeting, Boston, Mass., 2003.
6. Guyuron B, Bokhari F. Patient satisfaction following rhinoplasty. Aesthet Plast Surg. 1996;20(2):153–7.
7. Rohrich RJ, Janis JE, Kenkel JM. Male rhinoplasty. Plast Reconstr Surg. 2003;112(4):1071–85.
8. Wright MR. The male aesthetic patient. Arch Otolaryncol Head Neck Surg. 1987;113:724.
9. Slator R, Harris DL. Are rhinoplastic patients potentially mad? Br J Plast Surg. 1992;45(4):307–10.
10. Herruer JM, Prins JB, van Heerbeek N, Verhage-Damen GW, Ingels KJ. Negative predictors for satisfaction in patients seeking facial cosmetic surgery: a systematic review. Plast Reconstr Surg. 2015;135(6):1596–605.
11. Ishi LE, Tollefson TT, Basura GJ, Rosenfeld RM, Abramson PJ, Chalet SR, Davis KS, Doghramji K, Farrior EH, Finestone SA, Ishman SL, Murphy RX Jr, Park JG, Setzen M, Strike DJ, Walsh SA, Warner JP, Nnacheta LC. Clinical practice guideline: improving nasal form and function after Rhinoplasty. Otolaryngol Head Neck Surg. 2017;156(2):205–19.
12. Olley PC. Aspects of plastic surgery: social and psychological sequelae. Br Med J. 1974;3:322–4.
13. Wikipedia. Narcissistic personality disorder. https://en.wikipedia.org/wiki/Narcissistic_personality_disorder.

14. Zojaji R, Arshadi HR, Keshavarz M, Mazloum Farsibaf M, Golzari F, Khorashadizadeh M. Personality characteristics of patients seeking cosmetic rhinoplasty. Aesthet Plast Surg. 2014;38(6):1090–3.
15. Wright MR, Wright WK. A psychological study of patients undergoing cosmetic surgery. Arch Otolaryngol. 1975;101(3):145–51.
16. Zojaji R, Javanbakht M, Ghanadan A, Hosien H, Sadeghi H. High prevalence of personality abnormalities in patients seeking rhinoplasty. Otolaryngol Head Neck Surg. 2007;137(1):83–7.
17. American Psychiatric Association. Diagnostic and statistical manual of mental disorders. 5th ed. Washington, DC: Americal Psychiatric Association; 2013.
18. Edgerton MT, Landman MW, Pruzinsky T. Plastic surgery and psychotherapy in the treatment of 100 psychologically disturbed patients. Plast Reconstr Surg. 1991;88:594–608.
19. Picavet VA, Prokopakis EP, Gabriels L, Jorissen M, Hellings PW. High prevalence of body dysmorphic disorder symptoms in patients seeking rhinoplasty. Plast Reconstr Surg. 2011;128(2):509–17.
20. Sarwer DB, Crerand CE. Body Dysmorphic disorder and appearance enhancing medical treatments. Body Image. 2008;5(1):50–8.
21. Kyle A. Body dysmorphia and plastic surgery. Plast Surg Nurs. 2012;32:96e8.
22. Phillips KA, Wilhelm S, Koran LM, Didie ER, Fallon BA, Feusner J, Stein DJ. Body dysmorphic disorder: some key issues for DSM-V. Depress Anxiety. 2010;27:573–91.
23. Felix GA, de Brito MJ, Nahas FX, Tavares H, Cordas TA, Dini GM, Ferreira LM. Patients with mild to moderate body dysmorphic disorder may benefit from rhinoplasty. J Plast Reconstr Aesthet Surg. 2014;67(5):646–54.
24. Altamura C, Paluello MM, Mundo E, Medda S, Mannu P. Clinical and subclinical body dysmorphic disorder. Eur Arch Psychiatry Clin Neurosci. 2001;251:105–8.
25. Wilhelm S, Greenberg JL, Rosefield E, Kasarskis I, Blashill AJ. The body dysmorphic disorder symptom scale: development and preliminary validation of a self-report scale of symptom specific dysfunction. Body Image. 2016;17:82–7.
26. Last U, Moses S, Mahler D. Mental health correlates of valid perception of nasal deformity in female applicants for female rhinoplasty. Aesthet Plast Surg. 1983;7(2):77–80.
27. Nassab R, Matti B. Presenting concerns and surgical management of secondary rhinoplasty. Aesth Surg J. 2015;35(2):137–44.
28. Cerand CE, Franklin ME, Sarwer DB. Body dysmorphic disorder and cosmetic surgery. Plast Reconstr Surg. 2006;118:167–80.

Abbreviations

BDD   Body dysmorphic disorder
BPD   Borderline personality disorder
NPD   Narcissistic personality disorder
OCPD   Obsessive–compulsive personality disorder

9.1   Introduction

In modern society, more and more people report being unhappy with their appearance. In a US survey, 56% of women and 43% of men report dissatisfaction with their overall appearance [1]. This can be attributed either to the high standards of beauty that are promoted via mass media and social media or it may be an indirect manifestation of unmasked psychological disorders like depression and body dysmorphic disorder.

This tendency has largely contributed to the constantly increasing number of both men and women who resort to cosmetic procedures. According to the 2018 ASPS Statistics Report [2], 16.5 billion US dollars was spent for 17,721,671 surgical and nonsurgical cosmetic procedures performed in 2018 in the USA. This number represents a 2% rise from 2017 and a 163% rise from 2000. The desire to improve someone's appearance and get a better version of themselves is not even hindered by financial recession proving that cosmetic medicine is a recession-proof industry.

People increasingly seek cosmetic procedures, and someone would expect that procedures with objectively successful results would lead to enhanced self-esteem, better mood, and social confidence. In fact, the majority of cosmetic patients are satisfied with the results and consequently feel better about themselves psychologically [3].

© Springer Nature Switzerland AG 2020   79
P. Milothridis, *Cosmetic Patient Selection and Psychosocial Background*,
https://doi.org/10.1007/978-3-030-44725-0_9

The quality of the surgery and the surgeon's expertise are major factors that influence satisfaction, but they are not the sole determinants. In a retrospective study of rhinoplasty patients, surgery failed to satisfy 1.1% of the patients [4]. Dissatisfied patients sometimes, in the opinion of their surgeon and others, display objectively optimal results. However, they have no improvement in their body image, quality of life, and psychosocial well-being and occasionally suffer from deterioration of their psychological conditions.

Patient dissatisfaction also affects the physicians. When cosmetic patients are dissatisfied, doctors will suffer potential physical and emotional and financial injury. There is a significant psychological burden due to malpractice claims, threats, and verbally or even physically violent behaviors. An extreme paradigm is the case of assassination of plastic surgeon Jose Luis Vazquez and one of his nurses by an unhappy rhinoplasty patient in 1977.

Even if killing the doctor is not the typical ending of a case with unsatisfactory outcome, malpractice litigation is much more common. In a healthcare system that places emphasis on quality outcomes and harsher penalties for patient dissatisfaction, tolerance for adverse results and medical errors has diminished [5]. The high care standards of cosmetic medicine compared with rising patients' expectations often create window for malpractice litigation. In the past, malpractice cases were quoted to be responsible for about $10 billion in costs for healthcare providers in the USA [6]. Of those, plastic surgeons are more than twice as likely than other physicians to face at least one malpractice claim annually (15% vs. 7%) [7]. These statistics highlight the special challenges that cosmetic doctors face in their clinical practice.

A basic understanding of the factors implicated in malpractice claims can help physicians understand how to avoid common pitfalls. Apart from operative errors, bad communication when obtaining consent, deficient care before and after intervention, lack of empathy, and a failure to set appropriate expectations are likely to lead to lawsuits. Regarding cosmetic malpractice claims, patients pursued litigation because of disfigurement (42%), injury (24%), or psychological distress (9%) [5]. Apart from the objective complication of injury, disfigurement and psychological distress may occasionally comprise manifestations of the mentally unstable patient with unrealistic expectations who should be denied cosmetic surgery a priori.

The financial loss due to legal proceedings is also significant. The mean value of payout amount is 600,000 US dollars [5]. Payout is the sum of economic and noneconomic damage of the patient. Economic damage is characterized as the quantifiable expenses such as past and future medical expenses and loss of wages. Noneconomic damages are unquantifiable expenses relating to pain and suffering. Even though the majority of malpractice cases (72%) were successfully defended by cosmetic surgeons, the costs of correcting procedures, legal fees, and damages associated with psychological distress and lost wages are also significant.

Dissatisfied cosmetic patients often provide negative feedback at online review forums and social media platforms. A study of 1204 negative reviews following minimally and noninvasive cosmetic procedures found that the most common reason for patient dissatisfaction was ineffectiveness ($n = 782$, 65%) [8]. Having had complications is the second reason for negatively reviewing ($n = 301$, 25%). The abstract term "ineffectiveness" may conceal great expectations that were not achieved. Negative reviews are also significant psychological burden and an indirect cause of financial loss.

Cosmetic physicians' task to guarantee postoperative satisfaction for as much of their patients warrants the need to develop their skills to properly select their patients. In their office, they counsel a diversity of patients with various psychosocial characteristics. Above all, they have to manage patients' expectations to assure that they will ultimately benefit from the procedures.

There are certain characteristics that influence postoperative satisfaction and any improvement in quality of life and body image. These patients' characteristics are defined as "red flags" and should be taken into consideration by the cosmetic physician during patient selection [9]. The objective cosmetic outcome of the treatment is of paramount importance; yet, the basis for patient satisfaction lies in their psychosocial characteristics. Even though there are differences from culture to culture, region to region, and period to period, there are some certain determinants which every cosmetic doctor should be aware of.

9.2 Value of Optimal Patient Selection

Physicians tend to constantly improve their clinical knowledge and technical skills rather than develop communication skills to understand better their patients' motivation and build the essential bridges for a robust doctor–patient relationship. Interestingly, the educational program of most medical schools lacks courses and lessons about cosmetic patient selection.

However, in their everyday clinical practice, cosmetic physicians have the difficult task to identify candidates for an aesthetic procedure who are at high risk for an unfavorable outcome. Patients with psychological disturbances often present a concealed presentation of their condition at the first visit in the office. Disorders often come in various shades of gray and in varying degrees of intensity. This makes patient selection even more challenging.

A systematic review and meta-analysis examined 11 prospective studies, two retrospective studies, and one case study regarding the negative predictors for postoperative satisfaction [9]. This kind of knowledge is valuable for the cosmetic physicians in order to have happy patients and protect themselves from psychological distress and financial loss.

9.3 Predictors of Outcome in Cosmetic Medicine

The negative predictors for dissatisfaction following a cosmetic procedure are primarily separated in endogenous and exogenous factors. Endogenous factors are the unrealistic expectations about the outcome, searching for a secondary gain, and the history of various procedures to restore a feature in appearance or deformity, especially when it is minimal. Regarding their psychological characteristics, body dysmorphic disorder, depression, anxiety, and narcissistic, obsessive–compulsive, and schizotypal personality disorders and the "maximizer" profile negatively predict the outcome. Exogenous factors are the familiar disagreement with the procedure or the lack of consent by the husband or wife and manipulation from another person to seek and undergo the procedure.

9.4   Endogenous Predictors

There is a typical paradigm of people who are likely to have lower postoperative satisfaction following cosmetic procedures. This includes individuals with disturbed perception of their body image who tend to seek cosmetic procedures in an attempt to "correct" it. They may be worried even with minimal deformities and visit several cosmetic physicians to find the ideal one. Typically, they have great expectations about the outcome and even believe that their social and sexual life will improve. However, their psychological characteristics will not ultimately let them achieve adequate satisfaction.

9.4.1   Unrealistic Expectations

The most crucial determinant for outcome following cosmetic intervention might be the patient's level of expectation, which may or may not be realistic. Patients with high and unrealistic expectations have been described as "red flags" regarding postoperative disappointment. This factor is by far the most often described negative predictor for satisfaction [3, 10–16].

These patients expect that the cosmetic result will be ideal. They find it difficult to comprehend the unpredictability of human tissue and scar formation. They have the illusion that cosmetic doctors are magicians who can produce instantly recognizable results with no scars and minimal recovery time. If the patient views the procedure as a panacea for his or her life problems, the outcome is more likely to be poor [17].

During the preoperative consultation, cosmetic needs should be firmly understood and visualized. A handheld mirror is a necessary tool for the patients to better express their complaints and expectations and the physician to tell them if the expectations are realistic. Thus, perceptual inconsistencies are avoided [18].

Another useful tool for the cosmetic doctor is the 2-D or 3-D simulation software. Patients with unrealistic expectation often provide an unclear description of the aesthetic problem and find it difficult to express the changes they desire. During the simulation, they cannot suggest achievable changes, and when the doctor performs the alterations, they tend to prefer more radical and idealized changes. A mismatch between the surgeon's and the patients' expectations can result in dissatisfaction despite the outcome meeting a technical standard of excellence.

A special category of the cosmetic patients with unrealistic expectations is the highly demanding patients. They typically bring with them photographs of beautiful celebrities or edited photographs of themselves. Sometimes they even bring a pencil with them to draw the changes they desire and mark how many millimeters and what they want to alter. These actions should always be regarded with suspicion, because they generally cannot fully understand the unexpected nature of healing and usually demand a total makeover [19–20].

Consequently, patients' expectations about the cosmetic outcome should be thoroughly clarified during the consultation. Patients have to provide a detailed description of the changes they desire. 2-D or 3-D simulation software and handheld mirrors are used to start a conversation about the possible outcome. The conclusion of the discussion should always be the statement that the actual results may differ because of the unpredictability of the human tissue and patients have to fully understand it before undergoing the procedure.

9.4.2 History of Previous Cosmetic Procedures

Cosmetic physicians should be wary of patients who underwent previous procedures with an apparent successful result that was met with disappointment by the patient [12, 15]. They are called "surgiholics" because of their underlying addiction to aesthetic procedures. Goint et al. [21] excluded these types of patients from having a face-lift procedure because they idealized the surgeon and expected him or her to accomplish what others had failed to do. When "surgiholics" worship their physician during the first consultation, their declarations should be worrisome rather than complimenting. These patients also tend to make comparisons with previous doctors, always favoring the last one. Their deformity is typically minimal but is associated with excessive concern and maybe functional impairment.

These patients tend to be fully informed about the latest trends and nuances of procedures and have a fairly educated concept of what they expect the cosmetic physician to improve [19]. It may seem impressive if patients have a detailed knowledge about technical aspects and even anatomy. However, they do all this scientific search, because they usually struggle with a poor body image.

In addition to facing the psychiatric elements manifested in these patients, the physician is confronted with a more complex surgical anatomy because of the multiple previous procedures. Scar formation and anatomical changes make secondary cosmetic surgery more complex technically.

Thus, it is useful to routinely review past cosmetic interventions, including the number of previous procedures and their cosmetic and psychosocial outcome as perceived by both the patients and their family and friends. The cosmetic physician should be more concerned about people who have had numerous procedures performed by many practitioners and particularly those who report the outcome of such procedures to have been unsatisfactory. Any history of legal proceedings or threats is also obviously worrisome.

9.4.3   Gender

Modern men take care of their appearance as women do. They seek minimally invasive and surgical aesthetic procedures and desire to look fresh and young. However, they have been notoriously considered to be problematic cosmetic patients. Male sex has been described as a negative predictor of outcome regarding rhinoplasty. Gorney used the acronym SIMON (single, immature, male, overly expectant, and narcissistic) to describe potentially difficult patients to please [22].

Male rhinoplasty patients have relatively nonspecific complaints and are typically more demanding. They are also regarded as being much less attentive during consultation [23]. They tend to have more difficult time describing the changes they think are needed. When there is a tendency for selective hearing, a second consultation has to be scheduled.

Another study of male rhinoplasty surgery demonstrates that male patients seem to be more difficult to please than female patients. The younger the male patient, the greater the likelihood that he is dissatisfied with the surgical outcome. A greater number of males failed to appreciate any improvement in appearance compared to females [4].

Despite the evidence regarding surgical rhinoplasty, there is currently no data to establish male gender as a negative predictor for outcome following other cosmetic procedures.

9.4.4   Psychopathology

Merely having or having had a mental illness does not of itself preclude cosmetic procedures. However, certain psychiatric conditions may present with increased concern about appearance and are associated with poorer postoperative satisfaction. A detailed psychiatric history should be taken, and if there are any doubts, patients are referred to a mental health professional.

9.4.5   Body Dysmorphic Disorder (BDD)

The most notorious psychological condition that motivates individuals to seek cosmetic treatments is BDD. Unfortunately, patients with BDD generally respond poorly to cosmetic procedures. The clinical presentation is characterized by a preoccupation with an objectively absent or minimal deformity that causes significant distress or impairment in social, occupational, or other areas of functioning. People with this disorder are obsessed about the perceived defect, usually for hours each day.

In an attempt to alleviate their distress, sufferers may seek reassurance from others, check their appearance repeatedly at the mirror or other reflecting surfaces, pick their skin, and try to camouflage the "defect" using clothing, wigs, makeup, and hats

[24]. During consultations, it is not uncommon that in some patients the perception of severity of the anatomic feature they want to alter is disproportionate to the respective view by the surgeon. An individual with a minimal deformity but a high concern is likely to suffer from BDD and be dissatisfied by an objectively good result [25].

It is important to recognize BDD for two reasons. First, it appears that cosmetic procedures are rarely beneficial for these people. Most patients with BDD who have had a cosmetic procedure report that it was unsatisfactory and did not diminish concerns about their appearance [26–27]. Some patients end up to malpractice litigation or are even violent toward the treating physician [28]. Even though BDD is not an absolute contraindication for cosmetic intervention, there is a group of patients with subclinical or very mild symptoms who are satisfied by cosmetic rhinoplasty [29]. In any case, BDD patients should be referred to a mental health professional for evaluation before cosmetic intervention. Second, BDD is a treatable disorder. Serotonin-reuptake inhibitors and cognitive behavior therapy have been found to be effective in about two-thirds of patients with BDD.

Consequently, during consultation physicians have to rule out the presence of severe BDD symptoms. Excessive worries about a minimal flaw combined with repetitive behaviors are indications for further investigation.

9.4.6 Personality Disorders

A personality disorder is a type of mental disorder in which you have a rigid and unhealthy pattern of thinking, functioning, and behaving. Cosmetic patients who have personality disorders are possibly unsuitable candidates for intervention. Wright and Wright noted four psychogenic conditions that warrant special attention: "the psychotic individual" (schizotypal personality disorder), "the psychoneurotic individual," the one with "decisional disturbances," and the one with "inadequate personality" [30]. The inadequate personality includes the narcissistic personality disorder (NPD) and the manipulative controlling personality, also known as borderline personality disorder (BPD).

9.4.7 Narcissistic Personality Disorder

NPD is a personality disorder characterized by a long-term pattern of exaggerated feelings of self-importance, an excessive need for admiration, and a lack of empathy toward other people. They typically spend much time on their appearance. During the preoperative consultation, they seem to have superior expectations and do not really pay attention to what their physician suggests. As they typically bully other people, they may adopt this behavior toward their treating doctor, if they find the outcome unsatisfactory.

9.4.8   Borderline Personality Disorder

BPD is a mental health disorder of early adulthood that impacts the way someone thinks and feels about themselves and others, causing functioning problems in everyday life. It includes self-image issues, difficulty managing emotions and behavior, and a pattern of unstable relationships.

People with this disorder have an intense fear of abandonment or instability and may have difficulty tolerating being alone. However, impulsiveness and mood swings may push others away. They occasionally present self-harm behaviors, such as cutting. In cases of cosmetic procedures, self-harm attitudes will interfere with recovery.

The nine symptoms of BPD are:

- Fear of abandonment.
- Unstable relationships.
- Unclear or shifting self-image.
- Impulsive, self-destructive behaviors.
- Self-harm.
- Extreme emotional swings.
- Chronic feelings of emptiness.
- Explosive anger.

During the consultation, they may demonstrate extreme closeness and love (idealization) with their physician. Doctors should listen actively to BPD patients and be sympathetic toward them. They should not be operated without psychiatric consultation, because their psychiatric condition is likely to deteriorate after cosmetic surgery. As they tend to view things in extremes, such as very good or very bad, they may have a disproportionally negative opinion about their outcome. As they typically have problems controlling anger, inappropriate behavior postoperatively may also occur.

9.4.9   Schizotypal Personality Disorder (SPD)

SPD is a personality disorder that typically includes five or more of these signs and symptoms [31]:

- Being a loner and lacking close friends outside of the immediate family.
- Flat emotions or limited or inappropriate emotional responses.
- Persistent and excessive social anxiety.
- Incorrect interpretation of events, such as a feeling that something that is actually harmless or inoffensive has a direct personal meaning.
- Peculiar, eccentric, or unusual thinking, beliefs, or mannerisms.
- Suspicious or paranoid thoughts and constant doubts about the loyalty of others.
- Belief in special powers, such as mental telepathy or superstitions.

- Unusual perceptions, such as sensing an absent person's presence or having illusions.
- Dressing in peculiar ways, such as appearing unkempt or wearing oddly matched clothes.
- Peculiar style of speech, such as vague or unusual patterns of speaking or rambling oddly during conversations.

9.4.10 Obsessive–Compulsive Personality Disorder (OCPD)

OCPD is a personality disorder characterized by excessive concern with orderliness, perfectionism, attention to details, and mental and interpersonal control [32].

Surgical experience suggests that patients with significant OCPD traits may be more difficult to satisfy than those with histrionic traits, despite traditional psychological theories to the contrary [11]. Zojaji et al. [33] used the Minnesota Multiphasic Personality Inventory to establish personality traits in 66 rhinoplasty patients. Results of this study show that patients with certain personality traits such as "obsessiveness" and "psychasthenia" are possibly unsuitable for a cosmetic rhinoplasty.

The main symptoms of OCPD are:

- Preoccupation with remembering past events.
- Paying attention to minor details.
- Excessive compliance with existing social customs, rules, or regulations.
- Unwarranted compulsion to note-taking or making lists and schedules.
- Rigidity of one's beliefs (polarized: right or wrong with little margin between).
- Showing unreasonable degree of perfectionism.
- Obsessions with cleanness and organization.

9.4.11 Depression and Anxiety

Depression causes feelings of sadness and/or a loss of interest in activities once enjoyed. It can lead to a variety of emotional and physical problems and can decrease a person's ability to function.

Generally, it makes people to exaggerate the negative impact of events and, therefore, find it difficult to be happy with a result of any kind [34]. Preexisting severe depression can be unmasked after cosmetic facial surgery; on rare occasions, it even can manifest as psychosis postoperatively. These reactions tend to be more common after rhinoplasty than other cosmetic surgical procedures [35].

A study of 200 rhinoplasty patients which assessed various psychological elements before and after surgery revealed that preoperative anxiety correlated with postoperative depression, even without a negative effect on satisfaction [36]. Anxiety is a disorder known for excessive and unexpected worry that negatively affects daily life and routine. Psychosomatic research suggests that patients with high levels of body vigilance, health anxiety, or introverted temperaments may be predisposed to persistent physical complaints and excessive functional impairment when afflicted by medical illnesses [10, 37].

9.4.12 Maximizers/Satisficers

In the book *The Paradox of Choice* by Barry Schwartz, a consumer-based approach to analyzing satisfaction with a product is described [38]. The author identifies two types of decision-makers—maximizers and satisficers—based on their approaches to making decisions and the ease with which each experiences satisfaction after making a choice. Maximizers tend to be perfectionistic in their approach to decision-making and often experience regret after making the decision. Satisficers, in contrast, set acceptable criteria for themselves and will choose the option that meets their standard adequately. The maximizer–satisficer role model which is traditionally used in the product consumer setting may also be valuable in predicting postoperative satisfaction among cosmetic patients [39]. Cosmetic patients who displayed maximizer decision-making characteristics had lesser satisfaction with the result.

In the maximizer–satisficer survey, 13 items are involved. The more the respondent agrees, the more he approaches the maximizer role model:

- Whenever I am faced with a choice, I try to imagine what all the other possibilities are, even ones that aren't present at the moment.
- No matter how satisfied I am with my job, it's only right for me to be on the lookout for better opportunities.
- When I am in the car listening to radio, I often check other stations to see if something better is playing, even if I am relatively satisfied with what I'm listening to.
- When I watch TV, I channel surf often scanning through the available options even while attempting to watch one program.
- I treat relationships like clothing: I expect to try a lot on before finding the perfect fit.
- I often find it difficult to shop for a gift for a friend.
- Renting videos is really difficult. I'm always struggling to pick the best one.
- When shopping, I have a hard time finding clothes that I really love.
- I am a big fan of lists that attempt to rank things (the best movies, the best singers, the best athletes, the best novels, etc.).
- I find that writing is very difficult, even if it's just writing a letter to a friend, because it's so hard to word things just right. I often do several drafts of even simple things.
- No matter what I do, I have the highest standards of myself.
- I never settle for second best.
- I often fantasize about living in ways that are quite different from my actual life.

In general, presurgical psychiatric interviews are not accepted by cosmetic patients. In cases when a cosmetic physician suspects a psychiatric condition or a personality disorder, referral to mental health professional is mandatory.

9.5 Exogenous Predictors

Factors that have to do with someone's social network may also affect postoperative satisfaction. Family, lovers, and people from the working environment may increase someone's motivation to seek an alteration in their appearance. External motivation to have cosmetic improvements serves either as pleasing someone beloved or secondarily gaining something in professional or social life. In general, having an external motivation is notorious to correlate with lower satisfaction rates; thus, patients' motivational factors have to be clarified during the preoperative visit.

9.5.1 The Role of Family and Sexual Partner

Familiar approval is not necessary regarding adult cosmetic patients in terms of medical law. However, it makes things more comfortable if someone's beloved persons know about the planned procedure and approve of it. Miscommunications may lead to misunderstandings, and if there is a less than optimal result, it will produce the "see, I told you so" remarks, which will deepen the guilt that typically augments dissatisfaction [25]. These patients are usually obsessed about secrecy, hoping that their relatives or lovers will not be informed about the procedure.

Familiar disagreement with someone undergoing a cosmetic procedure has been found to be a negative predictor for outcome since 1974. Wright and Wright described rhinoplasty patients with decisional disturbances, as the ones who did not have consensus with their partner or family concerning the surgery [30].

Another group of cosmetic patients with decisional disturbances are the ones who hope that the surgery would improve their relationships. They may be falsely motivated that an alteration in their appearance will save a problematic marriage or improve other unfavorable interpersonal and social relationships. This is called secondary gain because the motivation has more to do with secondary thoughts rather than improving appearance. These disturbances are interpreted as an absolute surgical contraindication because the operation will be a disappointment when it does not lead to the relational improvement that was counted on [30].

Cosmetic patients also seek secondary gain when they aspire to improve their social or professional status with an alteration in appearance. Standards of beauty are usually thought to be associated with a happy social life and a successful career. People who undergo cosmetic intervention for these reasons may be frustrated when their expectations are not fulfilled in their social network. Thus, a distinction should be usefully made between expectations regarding the self, for example, to improve body image and expectations relating to external factors like enhancement of social network, establishing a relationship, or getting a job.

Another group of potentially problematic patients includes those who are pushed into a cosmetic procedure by someone else. They are motivated because of a desire to please a "significant other" or a relative, not because they want that particular procedure for themselves [19]. Olley also considered that these patients are contra-indicated for surgery [15]. He stated that a surgeon should not go along with the procedure if the request for surgery results from social pressure exerted by the sexual partner or family.

Thus, cosmetic physicians should always ask about the role of family and partners during the preoperative consultation and investigate any characteristics that may lead to negative outcomes.

9.6   Conclusion

There are certain psychosocial characteristic and exogenous factors of the cosmetic patients which negatively predict the postoperative outcome. These can be used for the development of a clinical tool for patient selection in cosmetic medicine.

References

1. Garner DM. Body image survey. Psychol Today. 1997;30:30–84.
2. 2018 ASPS Statistics. https://www.plasticsurgery.org/documents/News/Statistics/2018/plastic-surgery-statistics-full-report-2018.pdf.
3. Castle DJ, Honigman RJ, Phillips KA. Does cosmetic surgery improve psychosocial wellbeing? Med J Aust. 2002;176:601–4.
4. Guyuron B, Bokhari F. Patient satisfaction following rhinoplasty. Aesthetic Plast Surg. 1996;20(2):153–7.
5. Sarmiento S, Wen C, Cheah MA, Lee S, Rosson GD. Malpractice litigation in plastic surgery: can we identify patterns? Aesthet Surg J. 2019;
6. General Accounting Office. Medical liability: impact on hospital and physician costs extends beyond insurance. Washington DC: General Accounting Office; 1995.
7. Jena AB, Seabury S, Lakdawalla D, Chandra A. Malpractice risk according to physician specialty. N Engl J Med. 2011;365:629–36.
8. Watchmaker LE, Watchmaker JD, Callaghan D, Arndt KA, Dover JS. The unhappy cosmetic patient: lessons from unfavorable online reviews of minimally and noninvasive cosmetic procedures [published online ahead of print], 2019.
9. Herruer JM, Prins JB, van Heerbeek N, Verhage-Damen GW, Ingels KJ. Negative predictors for satisfaction in patients seeking facial cosmetic surgery. Plast Reconstr Surg. 2015;135(6):1596–605.
10. Honigman RJ, Phillips KA, Castle DJ. A review of psychosocial outcomes for patients seeking cosmetic surgery. Plast Reconstr Surg. 2004;113:1229–37.
11. Edgerton MT, Jacobson WE, Meyer E. Surgical-psychiatric study of patients seeking plastic (cosmetic) surgery: ninety-eight consecutive patients with minimal deformity. Br J Plast Surg. 1960;13:136–45.
12. Knorr NJ. Feminine loss of identity in rhinoplasty. Arch Otolaryngol. 1972;96:11–5.
13. Andretto AC. The central role of the nose in the face and the psyche: review of the nose and the psyche. Aesthet Plast Surg. 2007;31:406–10.

14. Tasman AJ. The psychological aspects of rhinoplasty. Curr Opin Otolaryngol Head Neck Surg. 2010;18:290–4.
15. Olley PC. Aspects of plastic surgery: social and psychological sequelae. Br Med J. 1974;3:322–4.
16. Rohrich RJ. Streamlining cosmetic surgery patient selection: just say no! Plast Reconstr Surg. 1999;104:220–1.
17. Beale S, Hambert G, Lisper HO, Ohlsen L, Palm B. Augmentation mammoplasty: the surgical and psychological effects of the operation and prediction of the result. Ann Plast Surg. 1985;14:473–93.
18. Gherghina A, Aristizabal M, Bay Aguilera S, Skopit S. Perspectives in cosmetic dermatology: what is in front of the mirror? J Cosmet Dermatol. 2018;17(5):672–4.
19. Gorney M. Recognition and management of the patient unsuitable for aesthetic surgery. Plast Reconstr Surg. 2010;126:2268–71.
20. Napoleon A. The presentation of personalities in plastic surgery. Ann Plast Surg. 1993;31:193–208.
21. Goin MK, Burgoyne RW, Goin JM, Staples FR. A prospective psychological study of 50 female face-lift patients. Plast Reconstr Surg. 1980;65:436–42.
22. Gorney M. Criteria for patient selection: An ounce of prevention. Presented at the Residents and Fellows Forum, Aesthetic Plastic Surgery Annual Meeting, Boston, Mass., May 16, 2003.
23. Rohrich RJ, Janis JE, Kenkel JM. Male rhinoplasty. Plast Reconstr Surg. 2003;112(4):1071–86.
24. Phillips KA. The broken mirror: understanding and treating body dysmorphic disorder. New York: Oxford University Press; 1996.
25. Gorney M. Mirror, mirror on the wall: the interface between illusion and reality in aesthetic surgery. Facial Plast Surg Clin North Am. 2008;16(2):203–5.
26. Veale D. Outcome of cosmetic surgery and "DIY" surgery in patients with body dysmorphic disorder. Psychiatr Bull. 2000;24:218–21.
27. Phillips KA, Grant JD, Siniscalchi J, Albertini RS. Surgical and non-psychiatric medical treatment of patients with body dysmorphic disorder. Psychosomatics. 2001;42:504–10.
28. Cotterill JA. Body dysmorphic disorder. Dermatol Clin. 1996;14:457–63.
29. Veale D, De Haro L, Lambrou C. Cosmetic rhinoplasty in body dysmorphic disorder. Br J Plast Surg. 2003;56(6):546–51.
30. Wright MR, Wright WK. A psychological study of patients undergoing cosmetic surgery. Arch Otolaryngol. 1975;101:145–51.
31. Schizotypal personality disorder. https://www.mayoclinic.org/diseases-conditions/schizotypal-personality-disorder/symptoms-causes/syc-20353919.
32. Obsessive-Compulsive Personality Disorder. https://en.wikipedia.org/wiki/Obsessive–compulsive_personality_disorder.
33. Zojaji R, Javanbakht M, Ghanadan A, Hosien H, Sadeghi H. High prevalence of personality abnormalities in patients seeking rhinoplasty. Otolaryngol Head Neck Surg. 2007;137:83–7.
34. Adamson PA, Chen T. The dangerous dozen--avoiding potential problem patients in cosmetic surgery. Facial Plast Surg Clin North Am. 2008;16(2):195–6.
35. Goin MK, Goin JM. Psychological effects of aesthetic facial surgery. Adv Psychosom Med. 1986;15:84–108.
36. Goin MK, Rees TD. A prospective study of patients' psychological reactions to rhinoplasty. Ann Plast Surg. 1991,27.210–5.
37. Sykes JM. Patient selection in facial plastic surgery. Facial Plast Surg Clin North Am. 2008;16:173–6.
38. Schwartz B. The paradox of choice: why more is less. New York: Harper Perrenial; 2005.
39. Oliver JD, Menapace DC, Staab JP, Friedman O, Recker C, Hamilton GS. How patient decision-making characteristics affect satisfaction in facial plastic surgery. Plast Reconstr Surg. 2019;144(6):1487–149.

Clinical Tool for Optimal Patient Selection

10

10.1 Introduction

Aesthetic physicians are exposed to risks not familiar to other physicians. They are the only doctors who generally are not trying to make a sick or injured individual well but, instead, make someone temporarily unwell to make him or her ultimately feel better, and the result will be judged entirely by subjective standards that are colored by self-image and illusions [1]. This situation becomes even more complex when one realizes that the degree of improvement achieved is only in the eye of the doctor.

Some cosmetic patients are dissatisfied with an objectively fair postoperative result. Doctors often tend to achieve clinical or surgical excellence but fail to develop their communication skills. Most patient dissatisfaction in aesthetic surgery is based on failures of communication and patient selection criteria and not on technical flaws [2, 3].

The ability to communicate clearly and well is probably the most outstanding characteristic of the claim-free cosmetic physician [4]. An optimal patient-doctor relationship is characterized by honesty, trust, and mutual respect. These three basic characteristics create an atmosphere for open and direct communication, yielding direct communication from both the patient and the doctor. Every aspect of the procedure and its complications should be clarified preoperatively. Any postoperative explanation is actually just an excuse.

Residency programs rarely include this field, but cosmetic doctors have to develop their communicational skills, as this will help them avoid psychological and financial injury from problematic patients.

Language barriers and cultural differences raise the need for extra attention. Every patient requires individualized examination and clarification of their motivations, goals, and expectations. This will diminish the chance of misunderstanding, leading to possible patient dissatisfaction and litigation [5].

Physicians do not have to provide cosmetic health care to any individual they encounter in their office. As Hippocrates said, benefit the patient, or at least not

© Springer Nature Switzerland AG 2020
93
P. Milothridis, *Cosmetic Patient Selection and Psychosocial Background*,
https://doi.org/10.1007/978-3-030-44725-0_10

harm them. However, there are individuals who will not benefit from aesthetic procedures in terms of postoperative satisfaction and improvement in self-esteem, body image, and quality of life. Daniel reports that cosmetic surgeons should never operate on an individual who they don't like, as the preoperative course is short term, but the postoperative period is infinite [6].

However, choosing patients according to someone's own subjective preferences would contradict common bioethical rules and medical legislation in most countries. There are certain psychosocial characteristics that are associated with poor postoperative outcome following cosmetic procedures. A clinical tool is developed to help doctors identify and select the patients who will benefit the most from cosmetic procedures. Patients who are excluded during patient selection should be referred to a mental health professional to investigate the presence of a psychological disorder.

10.2   First Approach of Cosmetic Patients

In most branches of medicine, "history" is an investigative tool, used as an aid in making a diagnosis. The diagnosis determines the treatment and its effectiveness; hence, most physicians develop their skills in taking history. On the other hand, in aesthetic medicine, the flaw in appearance is obvious, and the patients have a straight complaint about it. However, taking history in cosmetic practice is not meaningless. It assists patient selection, the importance of which was recognized as early as in 1968 [7].

People perceive beauty in a different way, and this may influence their motivation to seek a cosmetic procedure. Thus, aesthetic doctors should be aware of the concept of "aestheticality," which refers to how people assess human appearance. "Aestheticality" can be explained by considering a series of 20 pictures—the first a monkey and the last a beautiful woman, with each picture slightly different to its predecessor so that, over the 20 pictures, the metamorphosis is complete. Individuals' choice of where, in the series of pictures, "monkey" ends and "human" begins gives an indication of their "aestheticality." Those with a low level of aestheticality will accept various monkey faces as looking human, and those with a high sense of aestheticality will not accept "human" until all traces of monkey have disappeared [4]. Aesthetic doctors should be aware of their own aestheticality. This will assist them understand their patient's thoughts and motivations. They can also appreciate more easily the level of distress promoted by the appearance flaw or a postoperative result.

Understanding of patient's motivation and sincere communication with the doctor is the cornerstone for an optimal outcome. Research has shown that the most common factor causing a patient to sue after an unfavorable result is a breakdown in the relationship with his surgeon [8]. The physician must be concerned, understanding, and sincere. Emphasis should be given at the fact that they both have the responsibility for the decision to proceed with surgery and for the surgical outcome itself [9]. There is always a certain risk with any cosmetic procedure, either minor or significant, and it is patients' decision to undergo them if they believe that potential benefit exceeds any harm.

10.3   The Meeting Place

There are some certain rules that set the ground for an optimal first consultation. The medical office should be comfortable, with light colors. The background music is preferred to be relaxing, and screens playing loudly TV programs are avoided, as they may cause irritation. Waiting time should be kept at a minimal.

The interview starts with the doctor and patient meeting first and with a small talk until the patient feels comfortable. Greetings should be exchanged with a warm handshake, and the physician should look at the patient's eyes rather than any feature in order to guess the complaint [10]. An open question following the small talk could be: "What brought you to me?"

When the patient reveals the defect that he or she wishes to correct, the physician will look at it for the first time. Initially, there should not be any comments, but doctors have to objectively evaluate the feature. If the complains are about a body part, clinical examination will follow the history taking.

10.3.1   Is the Defect Objectively Significant?

In cases when the defect is absent or minimal, body dysmorphic disorder (BDD) should be suspected, and conversation should be guided to investigate this (Fig. 10.1).

Sometimes cosmetic patients are worried with imaginary flaws on their appearance. This state is called subjective dysmorphopathy. They overestimate a minimal or absent defect and become obsessed about it. Psychotherapy is the first-line treatment, and if obsessive symptoms subside, cosmetic intervention may be performed:

- A patient with exclusively subjective dysmorphopathy has a flaw that is only recognizable by them. This is the category of dysmorphophobia and it can be related to any body part. The therapeutic intervention is either psychotherapy or psychiatric medication; *no* surgery [11].
- Prevailing subjective dysmorphopathy stands for the condition when there is a deformity of the face or body contour, but only the patient and a low percentage of observers can recognize that. In such cases, cosmetic intervention may be performed, but adjunct psychotherapy is also indicated.

Therefore, it is important for cosmetic physicians to be aware of the anatomic norms and demonstrate the objective indications for cosmetic intervention. If the defect is objectively abnormal, doctors should ascertain that they have the technical ability to perform the procedure, before continuing the consultation.

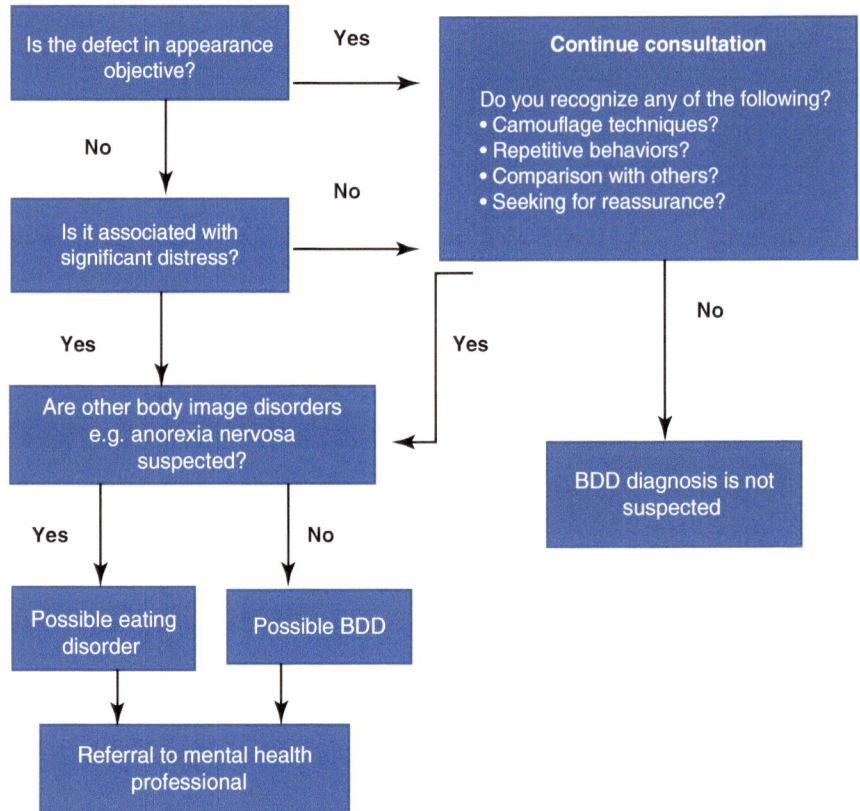

Fig. 10.1 An algorithm to identify BDD patients during preoperative consultation

10.3.2 Determine Patients' Sensitization

As a response at the question "What brought you to me?," the patient will report the complaint about his/her appearance. After that the history continues the chronological development of the symptoms [4].

Sensitization about a flaw in someone's appearance is the earliest episode that motivates them to seek cosmetic surgery, and it may be intrinsic or extrinsic. The first one refers to self-induced thoughts when someone looks at themselves at a mirror. Extrinsic sensitization is the result of extraneous remarks or teasing.

A patient sensitized about a feature on his/her appearance will scrutinize this feature on everyone else—always comparing and contrasting. Constant comparison with doctor's appearance may conceal stress in terms of body dysmorphic disorder.

If someone is not sensitized about a flaw of their appearance and seeks cosmetic treatment to please someone else, this should be recorded as it is associated with poor outcome. It is generally referred to as searching for secondary gain. Individuals who want to alter their appearance to improve their career and interpersonal relationships are potentially problematic candidates.

10.3.2.1   Useful Questions

- Do you believe that an improvement in your appearance/in the specific feature could make things in your marriage better?
- Would you feel that your parents/partner/children would treat you better after the cosmetic procedure?

10.3.3   Aesthetic Self-Assessment

Aesthetic self-assessment is the patient's own private evaluation of the feature of complaint. This is typically done in front of mirrors. The cosmetic doctor can use handheld mirrors to ask how patients assess their appearance in the bathroom. Patients are pleasantly surprised that their surgeon knows that this was done, that it is normal and predictable. At this point, they discuss about the improvements that are desired, and possible unrealistic expectations can be identified.

The most crucial determinant for outcome following cosmetic intervention might be the patient's level of expectation, which may or may not be realistic. Patients with high and unrealistic expectations have been described as "red flags" regarding postoperative disappointment. This factor is by far the most often described negative predictor for satisfaction [12–14].

Simulation software is a useful tool for cosmetic doctors to determine self-assessment and expectations. If patients cannot accept that cosmetic procedures' goal is improvement rather than perfection, then they should be excluded during patient selection. The software is used to demonstrate a realistic postoperative result and assess patients' expectations.

Patients with unrealistic expectation often provide an unclear description of the aesthetic problem and find it difficult to express the changes they desire. During the simulation, they cannot suggest achievable changes, and when the doctor performs the alterations, they tend to prefer more radical and idealized changes. A mismatch between the surgeon's and the patients' expectations can result in dissatisfaction despite the outcome meeting a technical standard of excellence.

10.3.4   Avoidance Behavior

Avoidance behavior patterns describe strategies employed by patients to camouflage or avoid exposure of their unwanted feature. These may involve, for example, choice of clothing, hairstyles, makeup, avoiding undressing with the lights on, sporting activities, positioning in front of a camera, and even weight gain. These strategies may conceal significant stress regarding the "defect." Their identification by the physician may lead to the diagnosis of BDD (Fig. 10.1). They should also be recorded as they should resolve following treatment and can be reminded to the patient as a postoperative benefit.

10.3.5 Other Important History Points

Cosmetic physicians should additionally take into consideration two points:

- **History of previous cosmetic procedures**

Cosmetic physicians should be wary of patients who underwent previous procedures with an apparent successful result that was met with disappointment by the patient [15, 16]. They are called "surgiholics" because of their underlying addiction to aesthetic procedures.

- **Familiar disagreement**

When taking history, a closed question should be made regarding patient's marital status. This could launch a quick investigation about the role of family or partner in the motivation for cosmetic treatment.

10.3.5.1 Useful Questions
- Are other family members aware of your plans to undergo the procedure?
- Do they approve of your decision to alter your appearance?

It makes things more comfortable if someone's beloved persons know about the planned procedure and approve of it. Miscommunications may lead to misunderstandings, and if there is a less than optimal result, it will produce the "see, I told you so" remarks, which will deepen the guilt that typically augments dissatisfaction [17]. These patients are usually obsessed about secrecy, hoping that their relatives or lovers will not be informed about the procedure.

The abovementioned evidence-based clinical tool is summarized. Cosmetic physicians can rely on it to carefully examine and just say "no" to those who are not likely to benefit from the procedures.

10.3.6 Referral to Mental Health Professionals

When cosmetic physicians are in doubt on selecting a patient for surgery, they should seek a second opinion from a psychiatrist or psychologist. This is also relevant when they suspect a psychiatric disorder that is associated with poor outcome following an aesthetic procedure:

- BDD.
- Depression.
- Anxiety.
- Narcissistic personality disorder.
- Borderline personality disorder.

- Schizotypal personality disorder.
- Obsessive-compulsive personality disorder.

Cosmetic physicians are not obliged to diagnose a psychiatric entity, but they should be aware of these common conditions and refer their patients to a mental health professional.

10.3.7 Selection of the Suitable Patient

If the cosmetic candidate seems to be suitable for intervention, doctors can proceed to discussion of specifics of the procedure, including all complications: operative risks, scars, change in sensation, possible asymmetry, and secondary surgery. Patients must realize that perfection is impossible and it is improvement that is expected.

The patient leaves the first consultation with a brochure of the data discussed. A second consultation is preferable to discuss again thoroughly the nature of the procedure, all limitations, and possible complications. It is then when informed consent is obtained. At the end, it clear that both physician and patient are aware about the suitability of the procedure and its potential benefits and risks.

10.4   Conclusion

Cosmetic physicians have a difficult task to identify the patients who are less likely to benefit from the procedures. This has to be performed preoperatively during a process called patient selection. An evidence-based clinical tool has been developed to assist doctors when consulting cosmetic candidates.

References

1. Gorney M. Mirror, mirror on the wall: the Interface between illusion and reality in aesthetic surgery. Facial Plast Surg Clin North Am. 2008;16(2):203–5.
2. Ward CM. Consenting and consulting for cosmetic surgery. Br J Plast Surg. 1998;51:547e50.
3. Gorney M. Essentials of malpractice claims prevention for the plastic surgeon. eMedicine. 2004.
4. Blackburn VF, Blackburn AV. Taking a history in aesthetic surgery: SAGA – the surgeon's tool for patient selection. J Plast Reconstr Aesthet Surg. 2008;61(7):723–9.
5. Vuyk H, Zijlker T. Psychosocial aspects of patient counseling and selection: a surgeon's perspective. Facial Plast Surg. 1995, 11(02)
6. Daniel RK. Rhinoplasty. Chapter 53. In: Aston SJ, Beasley RW, CHM T, editors. Grabb and Smith's plastic surgery. Philadelphia: Lipincott-Raven; 1997.
7. Grabb WC, Smith JW. Plastic surgery. A concise guide to clinical practice. Boston: Little: Brown; 1968.
8. Macgregor FC. Cosmetic surgery: a sociological analysis of litigation and a surgical specialty. Aesthet Plast Surg. 1984;8:219–24.

9. Wright MR. The elective surgeon's reaction to change and conflict. Arch Otolaryngol. 1984;110:318–22.
10. Goin JM, Goin MK, et al. Psychological aspects of aesthetic surgery. Chapter 1. In: Gonzalez-Ulloa M, Meyer R, Smith JW, editors. Aesthetic plastic surgery. St. Louis: Mosby; 1987.
11. Morselli PG, Micai A, Boriani F. Eumorphic plastic surgery: expectation versus satisfaction in body dysmorphic disorder. Aesthet Plast Surg. 2016;40(4):592–601.
12. Castle DJ, Honigman RJ, Phillips KA. Does cosmetic surgery improve psychosocial wellbeing? Med J Aust. 2002;176:601–4.
13. Honigman RJ, Phillips KA, Castle DJ. A review of psychosocial outcomes for patients seeking cosmetic surgery. Plast Reconstr Surg. 2004;113:1229–37.
14. Edgerton MT, Jacobson WE, Meyer E. Surgical-psychiatric study of patients seeking plastic (cosmetic) surgery: ninety-eight consecutive patients with minimal deformity. Br J Plast Surg. 1960;13:136–14.
15. Knorr NJ. Feminine loss of identity in rhinoplasty. Arch Otolaryngol. 1972;96:11–5.
16. Olley PC. Aspects of plastic surgery: social and psychological sequelae. Br Med J. 1974;3:322–4.
17. Gorney M. Mirror, mirror on the wall: the interface between illusion and reality in aesthetic surgery. Facial Plast Surg Clin North Am. 2008;16(2):203–5.